Healing Is For You!

A Handbook for Wholeness

Sandra Pavloff Conner

St. Ellen Press
Herrin, Illinois

FOREWORD

In the winter of 1993, Sandy Conner gave me a type-written manuscript of this book. She had written it to help minister to anyone in need of healing. At that time, my new granddaughter, Brooke, was seriously ill at the Cardinal Glennon Children's Hospital in St. Louis. She had been born about three and a half months prematurely, and we were asking God to move on her behalf – to cause her to live and to overcome a variety of present and potential health problems.

My wife and I first read the manuscript while we were in the waiting room of the hospital during an operation on Brooke. I would read a page of the manuscript and hand it to her to read next. We read all of it that day during Brooke's operation. The medical team had warned us of many potential hazards and problems, but even as we read the book, new hope began to well up inside of us – just concentrating on the faithfulness of God and getting a glimpse of His tender mercies. What an encouragement it was; what a faith builder it became! It ministered life to Brooke and to us as well. We began to realize that God's promises were real and that they were within our grasp.

What made it so helpful? Simple. It is soundly based on the Word of God, and I believe it was written with a strong anointing. Its purpose is to help the believer experience God's healing touch for himself and others. Frankly, it was never written for the purpose of selling books, but to be a valuable tool for anyone seeking healing.

Please understand that this book is one element, one tool, one effort to help achieve God's best. It cannot be used as a substitute for studying the Bible as a whole. It is intended to point the reader in the direction of the Bible – as a starting place. Think of it as a useful tool, but it must be used in conjunction with regularly studying the Bible, praying, giving testimony of God's truth, and reaching out to Godly men and women to stand with you. It is not a "quick fix" or an easy-formula short cut to healing.   Incorporate it into a well-balanced diet of all of these elements, but remember your main course must be God's Word itself. Feast on God's Word, digest it, and ask God to give you a hunger for more. Use *Healing Is For You!* as a resource and an aid to understanding. You'll find it helpful.

By the way, our granddaughter, Brooke, has had victory after victory in her first year of life. Serious lung infection – defeated; paralysis of her arm and leg – defeated; vision problems – defeated; physical coordination problems – defeated. At the time of this writing, we are amazed. Our church family is amazed. The doctors are amazed. And God is amazing. Brooke is a miracle of the Lord. What a testimony to the power and goodness of God! He *Is* Faithful!

Larry Bullock
Administrator, Christian Fellowship School
DuQuoin, Illinois

Editor's Note, 2017: At the time of the publication of this edition of *Healing Is For You!,* Brooke Bullock is a normal, happy, healthy adult who loves Jesus and gives Him glory with every day of her miraculous life.

ACKNOWLEDGEMENTS

I wish to express my loving gratitude, first of all, to **my late husband, Richard,** who was always my greatest supporter and earnest prayer warrior in my efforts to carry out God's call on my life. He cheerfully tolerated the upheaval of our home routine that naturally resulted from my taking out time and energy to write this first book, and he accepted without flinching that unenviable position of first critic of each chapter as it was written.

Secondly, I am most sincerely grateful to my sister **Dr. Brenda Calvert,** to my good friend and brother in the Lord, **Mr. Scott Boggis,** and to **Pastor Chris Hayward** and **Pastor Ted Pavloff**, all of whom gave generous and invaluable assistance in the editing and production of this book.

Thirdly, I offer my special thanks to **Mr. Stuart Davis**, whose constant Christ-like nature and servant's heart encouraged us all and faithfully under-girded the whole production process for the first edition.

Next, to my former pastor and loving shepherd, **Brother Percy Pavloff,** I offer thanks for which words are not enough. His vision for how much the Lord would use this book to bring the healing touch of Jesus to hurting people began the first time he read the unfinished manuscript. That vision was the catalyst that brought this book to its first printing. The anointing that flows from these pages is due in no small part to his consistent prayers and faith.

And finally, I offer my earnest love and gratitude to **Debra and Charles Funk.** Without their long-standing, unfailing encouragement and generous, practical help, St. Ellen Press would not be up and running and going strong, carrying God's truth to people who need it in all parts of the world.

God bless you all!

This book is lovingly dedicated to every sick and suffering man, woman, and child who will read the words printed on these pages. May you find within this book a God Who loves you dearly and yearns with all of His heart to make you well.

TABLE OF CONTENTS

Chapter 1: Jesus Is Our Doctor   1

Chapter 2: How Long Do You Want To Live?   21

Chapter 3: Inoculating Ourselves Against Hindrances   31

    Lack of Knowledge of God's Word   32

    Six Particularly Troubling Cases   32

    Unforgiveness   50

    Not Wanting to Be Well   60

    Looking at Symptoms Instead of the Word   61

    Failure to Submit to God in All Areas   68

    Possible Need for Deliverance   71

    Curses   77

    Lack of Ministry From the Local Body   88

Chapter 4: Means of Healing Prescribed in the Word   98

    Gifts of Healings & Working of Miracles   99

    Our Personal Prayer of Faith   101

    Prayers of Agreement   105

    Laying On of Hands   107

    Anointing With Oil   108

    The Lord's Supper (Holy Communion)   110

    Praying For Others   116

    Praying In Tongues   117

    The Word As Medicine   120

Chapter 5: God's Medicine Chest   133

JESUS IS OUR DOCTOR

Do you have a family physician? Is he kind, compassionate, and easy to talk to? Does he make house calls? Is he able to diagnose and treat all the various maladies that beset the different members of your family, without having to call in one or two specialists? Does he guarantee a complete cure every single time if you follow his instructions?

Well, the obvious answer to that question is a resounding "No" – at least if your physician is a member of the human race. No earthly doctor can possibly live up to those standards. But let me direct your attention to one doctor who does meet all of the above criteria. He's been in practice for thousands of years, and, as recorded in the book of Exodus 15:26, He hung out a shingle advertising His availability to all who have need of Him. He gladly takes on new patients daily, and He specializes in hopeless cases.

His name? Jesus Christ. Did you know that He is your doctor? Yes, the Almighty God who created our bodies and souls to be perfect, nevertheless knew that sin would invade our lives and with it the curse of death. Sickness, of course, is simply death in process. So our gracious Creator made provision for cleansing from sin and sickness. He shows Himself a healer at various times even in the book of Genesis, but in this passage in Exodus, He makes the clearest statement of all about His relationship to our need of physical and emotional healing.

1

When He delivered the Israelites from Egypt and began to make them a nation for His own purposes, He first established a covenant with them to govern His relationship with them. The very first covenant promise He made to this whole nation of people after bringing them from Egypt is in Exodus 15:26:

> *"If you will give earnest heed to the voice of the Lord your God, and do what is right in His sight, and keep all His statutes, I will put none of these diseases on you which I have put on the Egyptians, for I the Lord am your healer."*

Now, in the original Hebrew language, that word **healer** is literally **physician**, and to the Hebrew people, what the Lord had actually said was, *"I the Lord am your physician; **I am your doctor.**"* And isn't it interesting that, of all the needs a human being faces on this planet, God chose to deal first and foremost with meeting the need for bodily health?

A little later, He reaffirms Himself as the one who cares for His people's health, when He says in Exodus 23:25-26:

> *"You shall serve the Lord your God, and He will bless your bread and water, and I will remove sickness from your midst. There shall be no one miscarrying or barren in your land; I will fulfill the number of your days."*

You see, God never intended for His creation to be sick, because He never intended for them to sin. Nevertheless, He knew we would choose to rebel and give ourselves over to a cursed life. That being the case, He intended, from the beginning, to be the doctor for His people. He intended to remove sickness from them and cause them to walk in health and long life. From beginning to end, His Word resounds with promises about our healing coming from Him. Who is better qualified to do the job than the Creator Himself? He's a doctor who never loses a case that is entirely turned over to Him, and His prescriptions have no negative side effects.

Now, the Lord is not against us when we believe that we need to make use of human doctors or medications. Psalm 103:14 says that He remembers our frame, that we are dust. He realizes that most of us have been reared in a society, even a church society, that has, for centuries now, been taught that God doesn't heal the way He did when Jesus was here in the flesh, and that medical science is one of God's substitutes for what Jesus once offered. He understands that we must have time to let His truth create faith in us and set us free from those teachings.

God has His own means of healing, which we discuss in detail in a later chapter, but He is so concerned that we be well and whole that He is willing to work through any channel that we allow Him to work through to get us well. If we believe we need a human surgeon's hands, and if we pray, God will move heaven and earth to work through that surgeon's hands for us. If we believe we need an aspirin and pray over it before we take it, God will bless that aspirin to do us some good.

We must, by no means, belittle the human medical profession. On the contrary, most of the doctors and nurses that I have known have been kind, dedicated, sacrificing people. If it were not for them, many of God's people who have not known the truth about healing would have long ago been dead. And even if all believers looked only to the Lord for their healing, there would still be millions of non-believers who would die miserable deaths and suffer untold agonies if they had no access to doctors and human medicine. Christians who have a desire to enter the medical profession have a real mission field among non-believers for that very reason.

But beloved, as sons and daughters of God, we must always be raising our sights to God's highest and best. We need to be honest with ourselves, and each other, and recognize that medical science is *not* God's substitute for what Jesus once offered. Rather, medical science is man's best effort to help himself.

Dr. Herman B. Betten was only one of many medical doctors who, upon learning the full truth about God's healing, gave up the medical practice completely and began ministering God's Word and helping people receive healing through His Word and the power of His Spirit. In a sermon he preached in 1917, he explained why he gave up medicine. He said, "The reason I have given up the medical profession is not because I do not think it is a good thing, but because I have found something else that is better."
(Wilfred H. Right, *Jesus, God's Way of Healing & Power to Promote Health*, Harrison House, p.99).

God's people need to lay hold of that which is better. If we will stay faithfully in God's Word, apply it in obedience, and spend time with Him in prayer, we will come to the place where we are fully convinced that God has healing for us from His own hand. We will come to a place of faith that will let us receive health and life from our Heavenly Father and not have need of man's services.

God is the most experienced, most knowledgeable, best equipped, and least expensive physician, surgeon, nurse, and psychiatrist in the universe. He's the better way to health. We need to set our sights on His better way. We all know from experience that when driving a car, whatever direction we set our eyes is the direction our car will take. So it is in spiritual things. If we keep looking up – to God's highest and best way for us – we will rise to live on that level. We must not condemn ourselves for walking where we are, but neither should we be satisfied with always living with less than God's best.

So what should we look at? JESUS. Is it that simple? Basically, yes. We can hear all kinds of arguments, using Scriptures out of context, to tell us that God may not want us well, or that He may insist on our having surgery or taking human medication in order to get well. In truth, if a believer were to take those over-used Scriptures in the light of all the rest of God's Word, rather than the doctrines of men, revelation would come. I have often chuckled over the fact that so many who argue that we **must** use medicine, on the basis of Paul's telling Timothy to take a little wine for his stomach, are the very people who believe that it is always a sin to drink wine.

And I never fail to feel sorry for people who insist that Paul's "thorn in the flesh" was a physical illness, when Paul clearly says himself that it was an evil spirit – "a messenger from Satan" – sent to cause him problems in the natural. (2 Corinthians 12:7). Paul, and every Christian, must be willing to suffer persecution for the sake of the Gospel. Jesus didn't take that as our substitute. But He did take sickness, disease, and infirmity for spirit, soul, and body, so that we wouldn't have to; and it is an insult to Jesus Himself for us to choose to carry them again in ourselves.

There will always be arguments against believing God for our healing because, since the Garden of Eden, there have been arguments against taking God at His Word about anything. But as you, dear Christian, spend more and more time in the Word and prayer, the Truth will shed light on all those lies. (And this book does offer more detailed help concerning six of the most common arguments based on scripture passages that have been mistranslated or misinterpreted. You'll find that material in the third chapter, "Inoculating Ourselves Against Hindrances.")

So, does God Himself tell us in His Word exactly what to expect from Him concerning healing? He says in Psalm 103:3 that He *"forgives **all** of our iniquities and heals **all** of our diseases."* Psalm 107:20 says that when the Israelites were sick and dying as a result of their sin, God *"sent His word and healed them, and delivered them from their destructions."* The One Who forgives sin is the One Who delivers from its consequences. Are we saying then that sickness is always the result of sin? There may not always be a specific sin that leads to specific symptoms, but all sickness – death in process – is the result of sin gaining ascendancy over man in the Garden of Eden and bringing in the curse, which would eventually destroy all that sin had contaminated.

In Deuteronomy, chapter 28, when the Lord, through Moses, is instructing His people about the blessings of following Him and the curses of refusing to walk in relationship with Him, He lists a multitude of specific things involved in that curse. He names numerous diseases specifically, including mental sickness. But just so there won't be any misunderstanding, in verse 61, He says that all sickness and disease experienced by man are part of the curse of the broken law. But the great news is that according to Galatians, chapter 3, Jesus took that curse for us, and we now have become inheritors of the blessings.

So here we are, back again to Jesus. He not only took our sin so that we could be righteous; He also took our sickness so that we could be well. Let's read this same truth from another part of Scripture. Isaiah 53:4-5 (Amplified Version) says:

> *"Surely He has borne our griefs, sickness, weakness, and distress, and carried our sorrows and pains; . . . He was wounded for our transgressions; He was bruised for our guilt and iniquities; the chastisement needful to obtain peace and well-being for us was upon Him, and with the stripes that*

wounded Him, we are healed and made whole."

Now, does that really mean **physical and mental healing**? Let's be sure. Look at Matt. 8:16-17:

"And when evening had come, they brought to Him many who were demon possessed; and He cast out the spirits with a word, and healed all who were ill, in order that what was spoken through Isaiah the prophet might be fulfilled, saying, 'He Himself took our infirmities and carried away our diseases.'"

Could it be clearer, Beloved? Isaiah was prophesying a Savior who would fulfill all of the covenant promises of the Father God, including the promise to be the perfect physician for His people.

Notice that this prophecy, when translated fully from the Hebrew, includes griefs, sorrows, and distresses, all of which affect the mind and emotions. And if we will look at Isaiah 61:1, we find the picture of Jesus coming to heal the brokenhearted also. Jesus says in Luke, chapter 4, that He has come to fulfill the prophecy in Isaiah 61, so we can have confidence that there is no hurt or brokenness is our spirit or soul that is not also covered by Jesus' work. I can testify personally to two different times in my life when I experienced such a broken heart that I thought surely it was too shattered for the Lord to heal it completely. But, dear Christian, when I turned it all over to Him, He so completely healed my broken heart and restored my joy that I can barely remember how hopeless I felt. Jesus did that for me; no one else could have. He'll do it for you too.

Hebrews 1:3 says that Jesus was the *"exact representation of the nature of God."* He came to show us in the flesh exactly what God is like and what He will do. Indeed, He gives us such a complete picture of Himself as a compassionate, faithful doctor that if we will but look at it long enough, every doubt and fear will dissolve away, and we will have total confidence.

One of the main hindrances to our receiving healing is totally eliminated when we look at the preceding Scriptures. Many people feel that they have to talk God into healing them; they are afraid that it may not be His will every time. But an honest look at Isaiah 53, especially in combination with 1 Peter 2:24, which says, *"... by whose stripes you **were** healed,"* will make it clear that the Lord has already made His decision, once and for all. The question of healing is settled forever because God sees that work as having been completed and the price paid in full by Jesus. God's Word is settled forever in Heaven. Now all we have to do is settle it here on earth. We have to say, "I agree with you, God. Jesus paid for it. He's my healer. You said You would be my doctor and that Jesus was the fulfillment of every promise. So that means He's my doctor. I'll take Your healing."

Sometimes we look at the leper that came to Jesus in Matthew 8:2-3 and said, *"Lord, if you are willing, you can make me clean."* Now he hadn't had the opportunity of getting to know Jesus well enough to know for sure that He was always willing to heal. But you'll notice that Jesus didn't waste any time letting him know. His immediate response is, *"I will."* That settled the question, and that leper was able to tell people everywhere he went that Jesus was not only able, but very willing. Jesus' response to the centurion in that same chapter is equally as quick. As soon as He hears the need, He says, in verse 7, *"I will come and heal him."* Look at His willingness, beloved. He is so willing to heal – so hungry to meet the needs of His creation.

But, let us look at an even more wondrous sight. See the woman with the issue of blood, in Mark 5:25-30:

> *"Now a woman who had had a hemorrhage for twelve years and had endured much at the hands of many physicians, and had spent all that she had and was not helped at all, but rather had grown worse, after hearing about Jesus, came up in the crowd behind Him, and touched His cloak. For she was saying, 'If I just touch His garments, I shall get well.' And immediately the flow of her blood was dried up; and she felt in her body that she was healed of her affliction. And immediately Jesus, perceiving in Himself that the power proceeding from Him had gone forth, turned around in the crowd and said, 'Who touched My garments?'"*

Beloved child of God, let the picture of this event sink down deep into your spirit. See the brilliance of it as it outshines any other Scripture in expressing the finality of God's decision to heal His people. I can rarely think about it without tears springing to my eyes at the understanding of what our dear Lord has done for us. Examine the story closely, you who are still fearful that God may not be willing to heal you. This little woman had heard of Jesus. No doubt, she had heard many tell of His compassion, His wisdom, and His miracles. She may have even heard Him speak with her own ears, although that is doubtful, since she was considered unclean in her diseased state and probably would not have involved herself in public gatherings, except in this desperate hour. But she makes it clear by words from her own mouth that she has heard enough to know that this man is a healer. He has healing in His nature; He is so saturated with healing virtue that it even flows through His garments. She makes up her mind that she is going to have some of it, presses through the crowd, lays hold of Jesus' clothes, and receives complete healing.

Did she *ask* Jesus to heal her? NO. Did she ask if it was His will for her to be well? NO. Beloved, do you see? Not only did this little woman not ask Jesus to heal her; *she did not even get His permission* to take healing virtue from Him. Jesus Himself didn't know that anything was happening until He felt that healing power flow out of Him. Even then He didn't know who had received but had to ask.

"How could that happen?" you may ask. Well, God's nature is healing, and He sent Jesus to manifest His nature in the flesh. That woman saw that healing nature of God, accepted Jesus as the appointed vessel to dispense it, operated on her God-given covenant rights, and took her share, without asking. No need to ask. No need to get permission. God had promised, and then sent the fulfillment of the promise. His decision was made. He had come to set His people free from sin and deliver them from the curse. When a heart full of faith connects with the forever-settled Word of God, it's like striking a match against a hard surface: the result is inevitable. Hallelujah!

It would be good for us to look at another woman who recognized something in the nature of Jesus that caused her to know He could not refuse her healing. In Matthew 15, beginning at verse 21, we meet a Canaanite woman who has a daughter who is demon-possessed.

> *"And behold a Canaanite woman came out from that region, and began to cry out, saying, 'Have mercy on me, O Lord, Son of David; my daughter is cruelly demon-possessed.' But He did not answer her a word. And His disciples came to Him and kept asking Him, saying, 'Send her away, for she is shouting out after us.' But He answered and said, 'I was sent only to the lost sheep of the house of Israel.' But she came and began to bow down before Him, saying, 'Lord, help me!' And He answered and said, 'It is not good to take the children's bread and throw it to the dogs.' But she said, 'Yes, Lord, but even the dogs feed on the crumbs which fall from their master's table.' Then Jesus answered and said to her, 'O woman, your faith is great;*

be it done for you as you wish.' And her
daughter was healed at once."

Now this woman did not have a covenant with Jehovah as the Israelites had, so she did not have the same legal right to God's provisions of deliverance and healing. But she had a desperate need and had perceived something in Jesus that caused her to know that He could and would meet her need. Jesus does not speak to her immediately. Because He had deliberately laid aside His privileges as part of the Godhead to become a man like us, He ministered only through the anointing and gifts of the Holy Spirit – as He later instructs us to do. Throughout the Gospels, we see those ministry gifts operating in Him and revealing to Him people's thoughts and feelings. (Remember He did not run around reading people's minds. He spent hours in prayer so He could be super sensitive to the voice of the Father when it came to Him through the word of knowledge and the word of wisdom.) So I believe He was quiet at this point because He was listening to find out what the Father would instruct Him to do for this woman who had no covenant.

When He does speak, He reminds her that He was sent to the covenant people of God. Her only reaction is to ignore any indication that she doesn't fit the requirements and to continue to press in to get her need met. Then Jesus speaks more directly. He tells her that deliverance and healing are the bread that belongs to those in the covenant family of God, and not to those who are outside that family (who were often referred to as "dogs" in that day). He is walking out the ministry to this woman step by step, allowing her to recognize that she is not where she needs to be with God and allowing her the opportunity to keep moving into relationship with Him through her faith.

It has always seemed so remarkable to me that this woman could stand to hear such an answer and yet never waiver in her expectation that Jesus would give her what she asked. Jesus is so pleased with her response that He calls her a woman of "great faith," and He grants her request fully. What was it that marked this woman as being "great" in faith? She saw in Jesus the goodness and compassion of God, and she knew that could not fail. She ignored everything to the contrary. She would not consider any other answer but that this living God would meet her need. She determined to look **only** at God's loving nature, to press into it and hold on, somehow knowing that that very nature would not be able to refuse to meet her need without denying Itself.

In other words, she was asking Him to bypass rules and regulations and deal with her through His mercy only. Beloved, that kind of trust thrills the heart of God. If we will meet Him on the line of total faith and commitment to Him, refusing to give attention to anything to the contrary, His very nature and faithfulness to His Word will not allow Him to refuse us the help we need.

But, is that true every time? Well, let's look at the life of Jesus, the Physician. If, according to the Word, He is the only **complete** and **exact** representation of God and His will, then we will be able to tell if God is always willing to heal and deliver every person every time. It really doesn't take very long to read through the four gospels, and get a complete picture of the life of Jesus.

14

The fact is that Jesus healed everybody who came to Him for healing. He healed a lot of people who didn't come to Him, but He healed **everyone** who did come. Matthew 4:23 says that Jesus *"was healing **every kind of disease and every kind of sickness**."* Verse 24 says, *"they brought to Him **all** who were ill, ... and He healed them."* Luke 4:30 says, *"And while the sun was setting, **all** who had any sick with various diseases brought them to Him, and laying His hands on **every one of them**, He was healing them."* Luke 6:19 says, *"And all the multitude were trying to touch Him, for power was coming from Him and healing them **all**."* Matthew 12:15 says, *"But Jesus, aware of this, withdrew from there. And many followed Him, and He healed them **all**."*

ALL, ALL, ALL. There was never one to whom Jesus said, "No". There was never one to whom He said, "You'll have to wait." There was never one to whom He said, "I'm trying to teach you something through this sickness." No one seeking healing ever heard Him say, "I can't heal you because it's time for you to die." (On the contrary, He recalled several **from** death.) There was never one to whom He said, "Go down the street to Doctor So-and-So, and I'll give him the wisdom to give you an operation, and you'll get well." No, dear Christian.

History tells us that there was rather advanced medical science being practiced during the time of Jesus, and even as far back as Moses. Dr. Lillian Yoemans, who gave up her profession as a medical doctor to minister God's supernatural healing power to the sick, says in her book *Healing from Heaven,* "The history of medicine shows us that they (Egyptian physicians) had a most elaborate system of medicine and surgery ... The ancient Egyptians prior to and contemporaneous with Moses performed many surgical operations, including the removal of tumors and operations of the eye. As to medicine, they had an extensive pharmacopoeia." She goes on to say, "But the most striking thing about the attitude of the Word of God toward human systems of healing is that they are ignored therein as though they were non-existent. In view of the fact that elaborate systems of medical science flourished during the periods covered by the Sacred Record, it seems that no words could be more eloquent than the divine silence regarding them."(Lillian B. Yoemans, M.D., *Healing From Heaven*, revised edition, Gospel Publishing House, pp. 37, 38, 66).

Medical science was not a tool that Jesus needed to use. There are dedicated people out there today who offer medicine and surgery in an effort to help, but Jesus still has a better way. He can perform surgery without cutting into our body; He can perform surgery without costing us a fortune. Jesus never told anybody, "You go to man and get your help." Rather, He always said, *"I am your help. You can have it if you'll take it."*

God never changed His mind. He sent Jesus to destroy the work of the devil. That's why Jesus healed all that were oppressed of the devil. We never have to wonder if sickness is from God. God sent Jesus, and He healed every oppressed person, saying all the time that He was only doing the will of the Father. He's still doing the same thing today. How can we be sure? Malachi 3:6 says, *"For I, the Lord, do not change."* And Hebrews

13:8 says, *"Jesus Christ is the same yesterday, and today, and forever."* He has healing and deliverance for you today. If you're sick, make an appointment with the Great Physician, and let Him make you well!

Questions for Review

1. Where in Scripture does God first identify Himself as the doctor for His people?

2. Is medical science God's substitute for the healing Jesus offered while on earth?

3. In 2 Corinthians 12:7, Paul describes his "thorn in the flesh" as _____.

4. All sickness is the result of _____ gaining ascendancy over man.

5. In Deuteronomy 28, what is every sickness and disease known to man a part of?

6. What Old Testament scripture tells us that Jesus took both, all our sins and all of our physical sicknesses?

7. What New Testament scripture specifically fulfills the scripture indicated in the previous question?

8. According to Isaiah 53, when was the question of our healing settled, as far as God was concerned?

9. Which person in Scripture gave Jesus the best opportunity to make clear His will about our healing?

10. Which person in Scripture took God's healing power without even asking permission?

11. Which person in Scripture pressed in and held on for a miracle in the face of great obstacles, including words from Jesus that sounded discouraging?

12. Did Jesus heal everyone who came to Him asking for healing?

13. Did Jesus ever send an individual to a human doctor to get healed?

14. Name two medical doctors who gave up the medical profession to minister healing through the Word and Power of God.

Questions for Meditation and Discussion

1. What does the healing of the woman with the issue of blood tell us about God's will for our healing? What does it tell us about our covenant relationship with God?

2. Is God bound by His Word and His own nature to act in certain ways toward man, or is He free to change His mind and decide not to fulfill a promise sometimes?

3. Based on what we see in the life of Jesus, is it always God's will to heal? How does this fact compare with what the traditions and experiences in your life have led you to believe?

HOW LONG DO YOU WANT TO LIVE?

It never fails to grieve me when I meet someone in need of healing who believes that God has restricted each one of us to a designated number of years to live and that, as a result, we can't be sure if He wants to heal us when we may have come to the end of those years. They read verses like the one we quoted earlier in this book, from Exodus 23:26, where God says, *"I will fulfill the number of your days,"* and they assume that He has decided just exactly how many days that will be, and there's nothing we can do about it. But that idea is a deception from the enemy, and we can see this clearly if we will look carefully at the **whole** Word.

Again and again the Lord tells us that we have a very important part to play in determining how long we will live. To begin with, He says in Proverbs 18:21, *"Death and life are in the power of the tongue."* So, evidently, that which comes out of our mouth has great bearing on our length of life. Then, He also says in Proverbs 3:1-2, *"My son, do not forget my teaching, but let your heart keep my commandments; for length of days and years of life, and peace they will add to you."* The Lord gives the following instructions in Psalm 34:12-14: *"Who is the man who desires life and loves length of days that he may see good? Keep your tongue from evil and your lips from speaking deceit.* (There's that tongue again.) *Depart from evil and do good; Seek peace and pursue it."* This was such an important message that we find it

21

again in the New Testament, when Peter is moved by the Holy Spirit to quote these same words from Psalm 34 in 1 Peter, chapter 3.

Also in the New Testament, we find these words from Ephesians 6:2-3: *"Honor your father and mother – which is the first commandment with a promise – that it may be well with you and that you may live long on the earth."* Now, add to all these passages Psalm 91:16, which says, *"With a long life I will satisfy him and let him behold My salvation."* These several verses are by no means all the Scriptures on the subject, but they are more than enough to prove that the Lord has not preordained the date of our death and locked us into that time.

The other deception that many have fallen into concerning length of life comes from a passage of Scripture in Psalm 90. Beginning in verse 7, we read:

> *"For we have been consumed by Thine anger, and by Thy wrath we have been dismayed. Thou hast placed our iniquities before Thee, our secret sins in the light of Thy presence. For all our days have declined in Thy fury; we have finished our years like a sigh.* **As for the days of our life, they contain seventy years, or if due to strength, eighty years,** *yet their pride is but labor and sorrow; for soon it is gone and we fly away. ... So teach us to number our days, that we may present to Thee a heart of wisdom."*

So many people have read these verses – specifically the portion in bold print – and automatically assumed that they represent God's will and Word concerning how long we can expect to live. This verse has been quoted, taught, and trusted by millions as God's final word on the subject, until untold numbers of people in their 70's and 80's can't find faith to believe God for healing of their bodies and minds. They assume that since they're past 70 years of age, they can't count on anything more and may even assume that God doesn't want to heal them because it's their time to die. Nothing could be further from the truth!

We need to remember that Psalm 90 was not written by David and does not relate the promises and provisions of God which many of his psalms do. Psalm 90 was written by Moses and concerns the plight of the Israelites as they wandered in the wilderness as part of their punishment for their rebellion after God brought them to Canaan and told them to go in. They had sent in twelve men to spy out the land, and when ten of them reported that the men of Canaan were all too big and that the cities were too well fortified, the Israelites decided that they could not trust the Lord to fight for them and give them the land as He had promised. They refused to go in; rather they stood around and moaned and wailed and complained that they would all now die right there in the wilderness.

So the Lord spoke to them and told them that, because of their refusal to believe and obey Him, they would have what they **did** believe for and exactly what they had said out of their own mouths – that they would die right there in the wilderness. So they continued to wander there until their whole generation had died (except for Joshua and Caleb, who had believed God). They were indeed dying at the age of 70 or 80 because they were under a self-spoken curse, brought on by rebellion against God. If one reads the whole Psalm carefully, the picture is perfectly clear.

These words have nothing to do with the life span of the New Covenant man – the man in Jesus Christ – for whom the law of the Spirit of life in Christ Jesus has overcome the law of sin and death. Dear senior citizen, don't let false teaching, using this verse, rob you of faith for healing. Take these other verses that you **know** are God's promises. Plant them in your heart and expect your Lord to heal you in spirit, soul, and body – no matter what your age.

It's interesting to note that the Lord makes a statement in Genesis 6:3 concerning the length of man's days. Up to this time, men, especially those who walked with God, had commonly lived up to 600, 700, or 800 years. One can see that it took the curse a long time to actually kill man physically, but now, after almost 5,000 years of that curse in operation, we seem to be dropping like flies. Here in Genesis, the Lord is preparing to destroy all life (except Noah and his family) because they have all forsaken God, and we find this statement in verse 3: *"Then the Lord said, 'My Spirit shall not strive with man forever, because he also is flesh; nevertheless his days shall be one hundred and twenty years.'"*

Many people have wondered if this statement meant that God intended men to live to 120 years of age after the flood. I was especially interested recently in two different secular media reports concerning scientific studies of the human body and its cellular reproduction that seemed to focus on this question. The scientists concluded in these studies that the human body has a built-in biological clock that, if allowed to run its full sequence, would run 120 years.

One study, reported via national television news, indicated that if the body could function as it is seemingly intended to, there is no reason why it should wear out before 120 years of age. The other study, reported in the November 12, 1990 issue of *Time* magazine, looked at the other side of this truth. Researchers in this study proved that there is also a biological **upper limit** programmed into human cells, and, while the body should be able to live **to** 120 years, their evidence says that no human body is equipped to live **past** 120 years, regardless of medical advances that may eliminate most fatal diseases. Now, to be sure, a very few people have exceeded this age span, but according to this report, they are the exception.

However, a more thorough study of God's Word shows us that even after the flood, men were living hundreds of years before succumbing to the ravages of aging and disease. So that tells us that God's reference to 120 years was not His way of setting that age as a limit to man's length of life. And, in fact, it seems to me that, under a better covenant, at least some of us should be matching our Old Covenant forefathers year for year.

So why do we die at all? Because there's a spiritual law in effect that the Word calls "the law of sin and death." When sin came into the world, it brought forth a curse, including all sickness and disease, which destroys our bodies and shortens our lifetime on earth. Many

Christians believe that any time a believer dies, it is because God decided to take him. They believe that because Jesus, in Revelation 1:18, said, *" ... I hold the keys of death and Hades."* that He meant that from now on, no one would die unless He willed it. No, dear Christian. In the first place, God's will has never been, and never will be, death for His people. Ezekiel 18:32 tells us that God has no pleasure in the death of any of His creation. But death is part of the curse, and eventually comes to each person, bringing his or her stay on earth to a close. (The only exception to this experience will be the rapture of the Church when Jesus returns.)

It is because death is so repulsive to the Lord Himself that He had to win victory over it for His beloved children. When Jesus says He now has the keys of death, He means that death can no longer hold us locked in its grip. Before Jesus' finished work, the dead went to a waiting place often referred to as Hades – one part of which was comfortingly called Abraham's Bosom. Here, according to Luke, chapter 16, those who died in covenant with God rested, while those outside of that covenant suffered torment. Regardless of which side they were in, they were still eternally separated from God because they were unregenerate sinners.

Now Jesus has conquered the power of sin and the spiritual death that separates man from a holy God for eternity. That's why He was able to go into Hades, release those who believed, and take them into the Father's presence. He has not yet put the complete end to physical death, occurring when the spirit leaves the flesh, but He has secured the keys and has swung the prison door wide open, so that death now has no power or authority **to hold us**.

Jesus tells us in John 10:10 that He came to bring life, but the enemy is the one who kills, steals from, and destroys God's creation. St. Paul tells us in 1 Corinthians 11:29-30 that many were dying, not because it was the Lord's will, but because they were not judging themselves or discerning the Lord's body and blood in their celebration of the Lord's Supper. When the faithful Dorcas became sick and died, in Acts, chapter 9, the believers called for Peter. He did not say, "Accept this death as the Lord's will." Rather, he prayed for her and raised her from the dead. Also, when Paul preached past midnight and the young man fell from the window to his death, as recorded in Acts, chapter 20, Paul did not say, "Well, God wanted to take him home." No, beloved, he hurried down to him and raised him from the dead.

As we said earlier, God promised us a **long** life on this earth if we walk in covenant with Him. So, any death that cuts short a long life, or any death that occurs as the result of something included in the curse of the broken law (disease, miscarriage, enemy attack, accidents, etc.), is not the work or choice of God. He does not need to use such horrifying, mutilating, dehumanizing tactics to call His precious people home.

Many people have the mistaken idea that we cannot ever die if we do not get sick. Nonsense. God's plan for His children, beloved, is to give them health and usefulness all the time they are on this earth. When they are ready to come home to Him, He has only to withdraw the breath that He breathed into them, and they slip away to Heaven. Many of the saints of the Bible believed the

Lord for that health and fell asleep in Him when the time came to go home. Many of the saints of the twentieth century have done the same.

Remember, Psalm 91 says that if we'll dwell in the secret place of the Most High, He'll satisfy us with long life. Now that won't be a life of physical illness and agony, because that wouldn't be satisfying. That will be a life of health, strength, and fruitfulness. Psalm 92:14 says of the righteous, *"They will still yield fruit in old age."* And Job 5:26 says of the man who walks with God, *"You will come to the grave in full vigor, like the stacking of grain in its season."* We don't have to be sick to leave this life and go on to be with the Lord in Heaven. So, dear Believer, even if you're past 70 or 80, if you need healing, take it and go on yielding fruit for God!

Questions for Review

1. According to the Scriptures presented in this chapter, has God designated a specific date for each person's life to end?

2. List two Scriptures that tell us something we can do or fail to do that will affect our length of life.

3. Psalm 90 speaks of people living 70 or 80 years. What people is this Psalm referring to?

4. In Genesis 6:3, what does God say about how long man should live?

5. Have recent discoveries in medical science agreed or disagreed with Genesis 6:3?

6. People die because there is a spiritual law in effect in this world. What does the Word of God call that law?

7. According to Jesus, who is the only one who kills, steals, and destroys?

8. Name two instances when the Lord showed that death is not His will by raising someone from death.

9. Has God promised His people long life? Give two references that support your answer.

10. Do we have to be sick to die?

Questions for Meditation and Discussion

1. Jesus now holds the keys of death and hell. What does that really mean for us? Is death a servant of God or an enemy of God?

2. What can you tell someone who is past the age of 80 about believing God for healing?

INOCULATING OURSELVES
AGAINST HINDRANCES

Once we are convinced that the Lord really wants us well, we naturally have questions when we see Christians who aren't healed. "Why not?" we ask. "Why isn't everyone healed every time?" Well, dear Christian, there are many reasons, but none of them on God's account.

First of all, we need to establish in our hearts the truth that we cannot look at other people and their experiences of failure and make them our basis for faith. Any time a circumstance in the natural shows us something that is directly opposite to what Jesus continuously showed us in His living example of God's will, we must assume that the natural circumstance is not God's perfect will.

Most all believers have prayed for someone who did not get well. The temptation at those times is often to condemn the sick one or ourselves. To be sure, we need to be humble enough to go to the Lord and His Word and allow Him to show us if there's a hindrance we need to eliminate, but it is fruitless to continually beat ourselves down or to demand explanations from the Lord.

It isn't always our business why someone else does or does not receive something from God. Our business is to know that God's perfect will is healing and to act accordingly. Many times, we will just have to be satisfied with knowing what Jesus says about healing and looking only at Him. However, there are several

31

common hindrances to receiving our healing from the Lord, and perhaps, by looking at them in light of the Word, we can avoid them or learn how to overcome them.

Lack of Knowledge of God's Word

We might say that all of the other hindrances to healing are, in a way, outgrowths of this first one. Only a thorough knowledge of the Lord's Word, which is His will, can put us in a position to receive what we need from Him in any area.

We must study His Word, meditate His Word, pray His Word; and it will work for us every time. As a matter of fact, that very Word will itself give us revelation of possible hindrances in our life that could interfere with our receiving from God and show us how to deal with them.

We may be able to get healed sometimes entirely on someone else's faith or their ministry in the gifts of the Spirit, but the only way to be sure of receiving healing every single time, or of walking in health all the time, is to absolutely know the Word – and, thereby, absolutely know God Himself.

Six Particularly Troubling Cases

During my fifty years of ministry, I've come to realize that there are basically six specific cases in God's

Word where a need for deliverance or healing has brought about situations that have been totally misunderstood. The lives of each one of the individuals involved in those cases have their own unique aspects that, when taken out of context or from erroneous translations, can cause confusion.

Moreover, most of these cases have been made more troubling for Christians because some Bible teachers and some church denominations have chosen to interpret the scriptures focused on these cases on the basis of their own human reasoning and not on the basis of accurate translation of the scriptures themselves. For that reason, I have included discussion of these cases as part of the hindrance of failing to know and understand God's Word.

Case # 1: Job's Physical Suffering:

We'll begin with the case that most of the world — both Christians and non-Christians — are familiar with. I'm tempted to share here a lot more material than I'm going to let myself share. The book of Job has multi-faceted translation problems that can be cleared up easily when we take a good strong look at the Hebrew meanings of many of the words and phrases in that book. And Job's weaknesses and sins contributed significantly to his situation as well, but that subject too, can fill a book all by itself. In fact, I have written such a book, and I'd like to suggest that if you're reading this chapter and would like more detailed information about Job beyond what I'm going to share in the following few paragraphs, you can refer to the book *The Lord Giveth; The Devil Taketh Away*. The book is on the market, but is also available for free reading at the following website:

hanginoutwithgod.wordpress.com.

Most Bible students read the book of Job with the preconceived understanding that has been handed down to them for generations. They miss the all-important point of Scripture as a whole – that it all points to Jesus Christ, who says Himself that He is the only true picture of God the Father. Other scriptures verify that truth: John chapter 1 tells us that no one has known the Father, except the Only-Begotten Son, and He has come to reveal Him to us. Hebrews chapter 3 also tells us that Jesus is the *only exact representation* of the Father.

That being the case, we should automatically understand that unless a scripture passage lines up with Jesus and what He said and did, then that scripture has a problem in the translation or interpretation. Moreover, we are called upon by the words of 2 Timothy 2:15 to be sure that we learn to "rightly divide" the Word of God, and that includes knowing when the words we're reading are telling us what is in God's own heart as part of His covenant relationship with us, His children, and when the words we're reading are simply reporting to us what someone else said or did. The whole Word of God is true. But some passages are the Truths of our covenant, and others are truly reported words, thoughts, and actions of people other than God.

So let's first look at Job, who is described in chapter 1, verse 1 of our modern translations as being "perfect and upright." Now the word "perfect" in Hebrew has more than one meaning. It can mean that someone or something is complete or whole, or it can mean that he is without any fault or sin. Since the New Testament always sheds light on the Old, and we know from Romans 3:10 and 23 that there has never been a human being on the earth other than Jesus who never sinned, then we must conclude that the word "perfect" when referring to Job cannot mean that he was without sin or fault.

The only definition remaining is that Job was complete in his devotion to God. And he evidently was – to the best of his knowledge. But then we have to remember that he was living in a world of darkness – in the domain of Satan, who ruled the earth at that time – and that Job had no covenant with God to depend on for deliverance from Satan and his forces.

Job did have a hedge around him, but he tore that hedge down by his own fears. I will refrain from detailed examples of those fears, for the sake of time and space in this book, but I do cover them in the book on Job that I referred to earlier. Suffice it to say that Job himself declares that everything that happened to him was something that he had "greatly feared." That fear opened the door to everything Satan wanted to do.

The other problem we see with the book of Job has to do with Satan's approach to God concerning Job. Satan wants to cause Job trouble, and technically, Job is in Satan's domain (God acknowledges, "Behold, he is in your hand/domain.") But God asks Satan a question that is generally mistranslated as well. Modern translations have God asking Satan, "Have you considered my servant Job?" But that attitude of God – as if He's deliberating bating Satan to try to get him to test Job – does not line up with what we see in Jesus at all. Therefore, that can't be the correct translation of God's attitude in this conversation. But the literal Hebrew in this verse also has this following meaning: "Have you set your heart on my servant Job?"

Now, that changes the picture, doesn't it? What God really asked Satan was whether he had set his heart on having Job. And ultimately God has to admit that, because Job has no covenant – and because his own fear and his own pride have torn down the hedge of protection that had been around him – he is open to any attack Satan wants to inflict. But even in that case, God still forbids Satan to take Job's life.

Now we come to the third important truth about Job and what makes us know that we are not in a situation like his. When burying his children, Job makes the following statement: "The Lord gave, and the Lord hath taken away. Blessed be the name of the Lord." (Job 1:21.) Now, that kind of statement sounds holy. We use it at funerals all the time because it sounds like we're saying, "Even though God took my loved one away from me, I'm still willing to praise Him."

But, beloved Christian, that statement is totally without reason, and it is a slap in the face to God and to Jesus, who tells us clearly that what Job said that day was absolutely wrong. It's *truly reported* in the Word that Job said those words. But *those words are not truth.* Because

Jesus tells us clearly, "The thief cometh to kill, steal, and destroy, but I am come to give life, and that more abundantly." Jesus makes it irrevocably clear that it is not God who takes good things away from us. Only the thief steals from us – or kills us or destroys us."

So, if we look at Job through the correct understanding of that book in the original language – and through the words of Jesus Christ Himself – we find that God did not decide to inflict sickness and suffering and loss onto Job. Satan did it all – and only because Job had put himself into a position that left him open to Satan's whims.

With no redemption accomplished yet – and not even a covenant relationship with God through which he could get atonement and protection as Israel did once they had the Old Covenant in place – Job was a sitting duck – and God's hands were tied because He had put man in authority on earth – and only through the covenant with Abraham could God intervene and get things changed.

But hallelujah! Things are different now!!!

So if you're sick – or suffering anything else destructive in your life – and you've been believing that it's because you're another Job – you are wrong. You are not without a covenant. You are not in Satan's domain any longer. And you are not without a Savior who has paid for your sins and bought your healing with the stripes He bore on His back. So cast off that lie and reach out to the Father in Jesus' name and take your healing.

Case # 2: Paul's Thorn in the Flesh:

*"And lest I should be exalted above measure through the abundance of the revelations, there was given to me a thorn in the flesh, **the messenger of Satan** to buffet me. ... For this thing I besought the Lord thrice, that it might depart from me. And He said unto me, 'My grace is sufficient for thee: for My strength is made perfect in weakness.' Most gladly therefore will I rather glory in my infirmities, that the power of Christ may rest upon me. Therefore, I take pleasure in infirmities, in reproaches, in necessities, in persecutions, in distresses for Christ's sake: for when I am weak, then am I strong."*
2 Corinthians 12:7-10 (KJV)

Paul says in this passage that he was being plagued with a "thorn in the flesh" in order to prevent his being "exalted." He is referring to people exalting him as a way of exalting the message he was spreading. The revelation he had received concerning the Gospel was totally world-changing. As a result of that revelation, he preached that salvation is available to the whole world, Gentile as well as Jew. He preached the liberating news that all the world's sins had been dealt with by Jesus Christ and now the whole human race could be at peace with God. It seems reasonable, then that Satan, who is eternally lost, but not stupid, would pull out all the stops to try to destroy Paul and his message.

And Paul goes on to tell us exactly what that "thorn in the flesh" was – a **"messenger sent from Satan."** The word messenger in the original Greek means "angel" or "messenger." In this case, "angel" would have been the more accurate definition because this "thorn" was a demonic spirit (probably accompanied by several other demons). The Greek word used here is found 188 times in scripture, and 181 of those times it is translated "angel" rather than "messenger." However, the important point here is that it is *always* translated, not as a thing, but as a person – as a being with intellect and the ability to act and exert influence on others.

Throughout the Old and New Testaments, the terms "thorn in the flesh," or "thorn in the side" or "pricks in the eyes" are used to refer to personalities – either spiritual or physical – but never to sicknesses or diseases, or physical infirmities or disabilities. Paul, being an expert student of the Old Testament scriptures, knew the reference well – as did most of the nation of Israel, and that's why he used that term to describe the problem. The following passages are perfect examples of other scriptures that refer to personalities as being "thorns in the sides" or "pricks in the eyes" of God's people.

Numbers 33:55

Joshua 23:11-13

2 Samuel 23:6

Paul was not sick with a disease; he had no problem with his eyes (in fact he had shortly before this time received complete healing for his eyes after they were blinded by the power of the light that came from the presence of God on the road to Damascus.)

When he describes how the evil spirit caused him problems, he said the spirit "buffeted" him. That word means to hit repeatedly. Paul was being hit repeatedly from all sides by that spirit (and probably several helpers) stirring up people to attack Paul and to cause him danger on every hand. A sickness is not referred to as something that "buffets" an individual. However, spirits that stir up people to stone a preacher would definitely be described as "buffetting."

Moreover, when Paul says he will gladly glory in the problems caused by this messenger from Satan so that the power of Christ may come to the forefront, he describes the problems as "infirmities, reproaches, necessities (which means a lack of supplies), persecutions, and distresses." How honestly objective Bible students can turn that list of problems into an eye disease is totally beyond understanding.

Paul goes on to tell us clearly that when he talked to the Lord about it, the Lord told him that He had provided grace enough to deal with the problem and overcome it. This reference is similar to what James tells us in the first few verses of James, chapter 1, when he explains that in the midst of trials, when we commit to standing strong in the Lord, He energizes us with his grace gift of endurance, so that we can stand firm under any weight of attack and overcome it. Paul had that gift of endurance, and he also had the benefit of the nine supernatural ministry gifts of the Holy Spirit. He was well armed to deal successfully with that "messenger from Satan."

One last point, which should alleviate the final argument about Paul's case is the explanation of Paul's words in Galatians 6:11, when he says to the believers in Galatia, *"See with what large letters I am writing to you with my own hand."* There are scholarly treatises all over the place that supposedly "prove" that the word *letters* in this verse refers to the length of the epistle and other scholarly treatises that "prove" the word refers to characters of the alphabet. The problem seems to flare up for those who believe the word refers to characters of the alphabet. So let's deal with that possibility.

To begin with, Paul obviously is not referring to anything about a physical problem in his own eyes here because there is absolutely no reference or connecting words or phrases that would make that clear. If he was throwing in the fact that he is writing with large letters as a way of referring to bad eyesight, then he needed to make that connection clear. Paul was an extremely intelligent and educated man, and he knew how to write well – as evidenced by his exceptional epistles. He would not have just thrown in this statement completely outside of the context of the important doctrinal points he was making.

However, considering that he had just spent the whole epistle trying to explain to them the fact that Jesus' sacrifice had totally delivered the world from all sin and all the curse, and that now even Gentiles could become Abraham's offspring and inherit everything in the Kingdom of God, it seems only reasonable that he would write with extra large letters in order to drive home to them the seriousness and the power of what he was sharing with them.

As a writer myself, I have often done the same thing in letters, essays, and social media posts. So have thousands of other authors. Paul very well could have written with exceedingly large letters in this epistle to help establish these truths in the understanding of the believers he was addressing. But to assume that he did so because of an eye disease stretches the imagination far beyond the point of reason.

Case # 3: Trophimus Left Sick:

"Erastus remained at Corinth, but Trophimus I left sick at Miletus."
2 Tim. 4:20

Like many people in the Body of Christ today, Trophimus had been attacked in his physical body. We know that many times healing comes instantly, but many times it is a process that is worked out in our bodies. Evidently Trophimus was receiving a healing that was a process, and it was necessary for Paul to go on ahead.

We have no indication anywhere in scripture that Trophimus did not recover, so be careful that you do not translate Trophimus "being" sick into Trophimus "staying" sick or dying.

And most assuredly, there is not even the tiniest hint that it was God's will for him to be sick in the first place. The people who point to this scripture as an excuse for believing that God sometimes wills us to be sick rather than being healed are straining both spiritually and intellectually and still failing to make their point.

Case # 4: Lazarus' Death:

> *"So the sisters sent to Him saying Lord, he whom You love ... is sick. When Jesus received the message, He said, This sickness is not to end in death; but ... to honor God ... that the Son of God may be glorified through it. Now Jesus loved Martha and her sister and Lazarus. Therefore, when He heard that Lazarus was sick, He still stayed two days longer in the same place where He was,*
> *Then after that interval, He said to his disciples, Let us go back again to Judea. ... Our friend Lazarus is at rest and sleeping, but I am going there that I may awaken him out of his sleep. The disciples answered, Lord, if he is sleeping, he will recover. ... So then Jesus told them plainly, Lazarus is dead; and for your sake I am glad that I was not there; it will help you to believe – to trust and rely on Me. However, let us go to him. ... So when Jesus arrived, He found that Lazarus had already been in the tomb four days."*
> John 11:3-17 (AMP).

The entire event surrounding Lazarus' death and resurrection takes most of chapter 11, so I encourage everyone to read the full passage in his own Bible. However, for the sake of our points in this section of the book, I have quoted a condensed section of the verses that seem most necessary to our understanding.

Some people have been deceived concerning the scriptures in John 11 that give the account of Lazarus' death and resurrection. Scripture says that after Jesus received the message that Lazarus was sick, He waited two days before going to Bethany. There is an erroneous teaching that takes that fact and tries to make it look as though Jesus deliberately waited for Lazarus to die before He went to be with the family. However, a close look at the time frame in this passage of Scripture will clear up that misconception.

We know, from Philippians description of Jesus decision to step down from His throne and come to earth as a human being that He laid aside all the privileges and advantages of being part of the Godhead so that He could live His life of obedience as a human being without unfair advantages. That being the case, He needed the Holy Spirit infilling and His gifts in order to minister to people on a supernatural level. We've already discussed this fact in an earlier lesson in this book, so we won't elaborate here. But we see that supernatural "word of knowledge" operating in this passage from John 11.

In this case of Lazarus, Jesus received supernatural revelation from the Spirit that Lazarus was not only sick, but that he had already died. When he tells his disciples that He's going to Bethany and they argue with Him, He reveals to them that He already knows Lazarus is dead.

So, in fact, the reason He hadn't hurried to Bethany immediately was because He knew by the Spirit that Lazarus was already dead. Jesus waited two days before going to Mary and Martha. But when He got there, Lazarus had already been in the grave for four days. If we look at the time frame, it's easy to see that Lazarus had to have been dead by the time Jesus received the messenger who had been sent by Mary and Martha.

Jesus also explains to His disciples that He's glad – for their sakes – that they would be able to see an even more exciting miracle than a healing. They would see a resurrection and a healing all in one – and that for a man who had been in the grave four days.

But it was **not** Jesus' decision to **wait** until Lazarus died and had been buried four days before He went to Bethany. If that had been the case – if Lazarus had still been alive when Jesus received the message – then He would have had to wait longer than two days. So the teaching that sometimes God waits to heal us – so that our condition will worsen and the miracle will seem bigger – cannot be found in God's Word. It cannot be based on Jesus' actions concerning Lazarus or on any other of Jesus' actions when He ministered on earth.

The final two cases we'll look at in detail have to do with the erroneous teaching that God requires us to make use of medical science and not trust Him and His Word alone for our healing and health. We've discussed God's attitude toward medical science in the first chapter of this book, so we won't belabor that point. We'll just look at the two cases generally used for this argument and see just how lacking in evidence they are.

Case # 5: Hezekiah's Poultice:

There are two parallel accounts of Hezekiah's ordeal: one in Isaiah 38 and the other in 2 Kings 20. As with the account of Lazarus, the full passage is much too long to quote here, but I do encourage readers to search their own Bibles in both of those references for the full story. I'm quoting only the passages that seem particularly relevant to our point.

> *"In those days Hezekiah became mortally ill. And Isaiah the prophet the son of Amoz came to him and said to him, Thus says the Lord, Set you house in order, for you shall die and not live. Then Hezekiah turned his face to the wall and prayed to the Lord and said, Remember now, O Lord, I beseech Thee, how I have walked before Thee in truth and with a whole heart, and have done what is good in They sight. And Hezekiah wept bitterly. Then the word of the Lord came to Isaiah saying, Go and say to Hezekiah, Thus says the Lord, the God of your father David. I have heard your prayer; I have seen your tears: behold I will add fifteen years to your life. And I will deliver you and this city from the hand of the king of Assyria; and I will defend this city.*

*And this shall be the sign to you from the
Lord, that the Lord will do this thing that He
has spoken. Behold I will cause the shadow
on the stairway, which has gone down with
the sun on the stairway of Ahaz, to go back
ten steps. So the suns' shadow went back ten
steps on the stairway on which it had gone
down.".*   Isaiah 38:1-8

Verses 9-20 then gives a lengthy writing by
Hezekiah himself concerning his sickness and his
gratitude for being given a longer life to serve the Lord.
After that passage, verse 21 then adds these words: *"Now
Isaiah had said, Let them take a cake of figs and apply it
to the boil, that he may recover."*

The scriptural account of Hezekiah does not say
specifically what Hezekiah's disease was. We just know
that the Lord sent the prophet Isaiah to let Hezekiah
know that his sickness was mortal, and that he would not
recover. Be careful not to read into this passage that the
Lord "wanted" Hezekiah to die. There is absolutely no
support for that fact. In fact, since the Lord immediately
responds to Hezekiah's prayer with deliverance and
healing, we have every reason to believe that the Lord
sent him the warning so that he would pray and open the
door for God to heal him.

In the original ancient texts of Isaiah 38, verses 21
and 22 (referring to a poultice applied to a boil) do not
exist. Nor are they found in the original copying of the

text in the Dead Sea Scrolls. However, in the Dead Sea Scrolls, those two verses had been added between verses and written in such a way so as to extend into the margin of the scroll – because the words were not included in the first copy of that book. There are no ancient copies of the parallel story in 2 Kings, but it seems reasonable to assume that if the original book of Isaiah did not include application of a poultice, then it was not part of the factual story.

It should also be noted that in neither of the accounts does Isaiah say that the "Lord said to apply a poultice." Whenever Isaiah spoke words the Lord had instructed him to speak, he always prefaced those words with, "Thus saith the Lord." But when he supposedly commanded a poultice be applied, he did not use those words. So even if he did actually say those words, he was giving his own human interpretation of the situation and its remedy and not the Lord's.

Moreover, if Hezekiah's problem was indeed a boil serious enough to cause his death, then that meant the infection had become systemic and had spread throughout his entire body. Any modern medical doctor will agree that in a case where a deadly boil has caused systemic poisoning throughout the body, no poultice applied to the outside of the skin will draw out that poison enough to save the patient's life.

So critics of believers who choose to make the Lord their only doctor, actually have no legitimate evidence to indicate that the Lord required Hezekiah to use a man-made medication in order to get his healing manifested.

Case # 6: Timothy's Wine:

"Drink no longer water; but use a little wine for thy stomach's sake and thine often infirmities."   1 Tim. 5:23 (KJV)

Since the water in that area of the world was not healthy to drink, this advice was common, as was the practice of taking wine with meals. Evidently Timothy had not adopted the practice, so Paul advises him to do so. Doctors today tell us that drinking a little wine benefits the heart, as well as some other parts of the body. So Paul's recommendation seems little more than good advice for being a good steward of the body in that region of the country.

But even if readers want to believe that Timothy had some physical problem with his stomach, we cannot look at his situation to determine God's will for our health. We do not know where Timothy's faith was concerning health and healing, and we must never decide what to believe about God's healing based on Timothy or Paul. We must decide based on Jesus alone.

To be sure, there are other scritpure passages that sometimes stir up questions in readers' minds, but these six have been abused for many generations and have provided a lot of fuel for the enemy as he fights the truth that God wants to heal His people and keep them well as long as they are working on this earth. Hopefully, taking the time and space to consider all six of these troublesome passages will help alleviate the lies and the misunderstandings for you, dear readers. As you can readily see, these passages lose their power to cause doubt and unbelief once the Word of God is thoroughly understood.

===============

Unforgiveness

One of the most important hindrances to our receiving anything from the Lord by faith is unforgiveness. In the world we live in, it is so easy to get into strife and conflict. People say and do things that hurt others, sometimes unknowingly, sometimes deliberately. Moreover, our enemy, Satan, will do his best to cause others, especially people we're close to, to inflict wounds of various kinds in order to get us out of God's will through negative reactions, and thereby hinder God's work.

Needless to say, the subject of forgiveness is vast enough to fill a whole book all by itself, and obviously we will not even try to cover everything the Word says about it. However, we must settle it in our hearts that forgiveness of sin is the foundation from which all other blessings come to us from God. It is because we are forgiven that we can be healed. The sin that brought on the curse in the first place is put away, and then the curse itself can be eradicated. When Jesus ministered to the paralytic in Matthew, chapter 9, He first told him to take courage because his sins were forgiven. When the scribes got upset, Jesus answered them in verses 5 and 6 by saying:

"For which is easier to say, 'Your sins are forgiven' or to say, 'Rise and walk?' But in order that you may know that the Son of Man has authority on earth to forgive sins, -- then He said to the paralytic, 'Rise. Take up your bed and go home.'"

You see, the scribes understood that, according to their covenant with God, they had to recognize a connection between man's sinfulness and the curse, which included all diseases. They recognized that if the paralytic was healed, then that meant his sins had been forgiven. They knew that a sacrifice had to be made to atone for sin in order for the blessings of the covenant, including healing, to come to them. When Jesus came as the ultimate sacrifice, His finished work brought freedom from sin as well as the curse for mankind.

We're going to look at two passages of scripture in which Jesus makes very clear how the Father feels about our being willing to forgive others. He says in Matthew 6:14-15,

"For if you forgive men for their transgressions, your Heavenly Father will also forgive you, but if you do not forgive men, then your Father will not forgive your transgressions."

Then again, when giving those wonderful instructions about how to operate mountain-moving faith in Mark 11, He says in verse 25 and 26,

*"And whenever you stand praying, forgive,
if you have anything against anyone; so
that your Father also who is in heaven may
forgive you your transgressions. But if you
do not forgive, neither will your Father
who is in heaven forgive your
transgressions."*

Now, these two passages of scripture must be understood for what they are: insgtructions for living successfully under the Old Covenant. Once Jesus died for all sin and issued forth the "ministry of reconciliation" described in 2 Corinthians, chapter 5, the forgiveness from the Father shifts into being a finished work. You see, Jesus died to purchase forgiveness for all mankind, and that means you and me.

While it's not the purpose of this book to teach the concept of the ministry of reconciliation in detail, it seems beneficial to at least explain the most important aspect of it. 2 Corinthians 5:17-19 says it clearly:

*"Therefore, if any man is in Christ, he is a
new creature; the old things passed away;
behold nw things have come. Now all these
things are from God, who reconciled us to
Himself through Christ, and gave us the
ministry of reconciliation, namely, that God
was in Christ reconciling the **world** to
Himself, **not counting their trespasses
against them**, and He has committed to us the
word of reconciliation."*

Notice that God's definition of the "ministry of reconciliation" is that we are to let the whole world know that, in Christ, God is "no longer counting their sins against them." In other words, in Christ, all sin is legally forgiven. Now, of course, anyone who does not accept Christ does not walk in that benefit, and for those of us who are Christians, we still need to be aware when we sin and turn to the Father in repentance in order to appropriate that forgiveness. (1 John 1:9).

The point here is that God considers the work finished – the only worthy sacrifice (Jesus) has been offered for all sin – and the Father has accepted that sacrifice and granted complete and eternal forgiveness. He no longer deliberately withholds forgiveness based on an individual's behavior or an individual's sacrifice. Forgiveness is a done deal now – but available only in Christ.

However, that legal situation does not change the fact that our failure to forgive can keep us from receiving our healing. We must remember that God is Love. And God's Kingdom operates on laws that emanate from God's nature – the primary element of that nature being love. So the primary law of the Kingdom is Love, and none of the other laws of that Kingdom will operate the way they are intended to operate if we are in rebellion to the primary law.

Galatians 5:6 tells us clearly that our faith operates by love. So if we are not walking in love, our faith is not able to function at high capacity. When we refuse to forgive, we are outside the love realm, and our own hearts condemn us.

Moreover, when we refuse to forgive, we are placing ourselves above God in our own estimation. Let's face it, no matter how strong a Christian home we were brought up in, or how young we were when we accepted Jesus as Lord, we were all born in sin, and unless He had died to provide mercy for us, we would have spent eternity in Hell. He forgives, and, when we refuse to forgive another person, we are, in effect, saying we are better than He is; we are too good to forgive someone else's sin, even though He died to forgive them – and has forgiven us for all of our sin. And, beloved, when we put ourselves **above** Jesus, let us not think that we will be in a position to receive **from** Him.

If we're smart, we'll keep ourselves on a plane where we can easily receive everything we need. And, after all, we claim as believers that we want to be just like the Lord. That means we must forgive as God does. He forgives whether we repent or not; we just can't experience the forgiveness or its benefits until we come in confession and receive. So, we too must forgive others whether they repent or not. From our heart, by our will, we must make the decision not to hold sin of any kind against another. By doing so, we keep the channel open to receive from God, and we keep ourselves free from all of the destruction worked by the resentment and bitterness that go hand in hand with unforgiveness.

The destructive effects of unforgiveness can, in themselves, cause sickness and infirmity of soul or body. Doctors around the world have told us for decades that bitterness and unforgiveness wreak havoc on the body and open us up to many diseases and physical afflictions.

Don't be deceived, dear Christian. The Lord means what He says. When we refuse to forgive, we are refusing to submit to God, consequently taking ourselves out from under His protection. Remember, James 4:7 says, *"Submit therefore to God. Resist the devil and he will flee from you."* But, notice that we must submit to God first. Refusing to forgive is refusing to submit. Therefore, we are wide open for attack by the destroyer.

I will take the time here to briefly share a personal experience that I had concerning unforgiveness. I did not actually become physically ill, but my physical body was so affected that I was miserable. I had been terribly hurt by some individuals, repeatedly hurt as a matter of fact, and had at one point made a decision to forgive them. I thought I had settled the matter once and for all, but gradually I began to think about some of the things that had been done and said to me. I began to replay them again and again in my mind and naturally gave place to the hurt feelings they had originally caused.

I fell into the trap so many Christians fall into, in that I did not guard against consciously remembering and meditating on the once forgiven sins. God doesn't allow Himself to ever again remember or think on our forgiven sins, and we must be vigilant enough to recognize this subtle trap of the enemy. Well, I was not vigilant, and though I was not actually resentful toward these people for their treatment of me, I was actually being hospitable to the spirits of unforgiveness, resentment, and self-pity by meditating on the sins.

One day I noticed an odor like that of garbage after it has accumulated for a long period of time. I thought it was just something in the air, so I tried to ignore it. The odor continued with me all day and even at night in bed. The second day, I noticed it again. The third day was Sunday, and, even while in church, I was bothered by that distinct, abhorrent odor.

Each time I experienced this smell, I asked my husband if he could smell it, and he said that he couldn't. After finally getting into bed the third night, with the odor still pungent but noticeable only to me, I was distraught. A time or two during the process of this experience, the thought of some connection with unforgiveness had sort of floated gently into my mind, but I had instantly dismissed it, certain that I was not experiencing that problem.

However, the third night I told my husband that I needed prayer for the situation because I just couldn't figure out what was going on. He was in quiet thought for a few minutes and then said, "Do you think it could be connected with unforgiveness?"

Well, the Lord didn't have to hit me on the head with a hammer. I knew He had revealed to my husband what the root of the problem was. I hadn't mentioned anything to my husband about the thoughts I'd been having, so the only way he could have come up with that idea was from the Lord. Of course, the Lord had been trying for a couple days to tell me what was happening, but I guess I didn't really want to acknowledge that I had slipped back into unforgiveness.

Needless to say, My husband and I prayed immediately. I repented, first of all, for picking back up someone's old sins that had been put away and for allowing those nasty spirits to feed their thoughts and feelings of resentment and self-pity into me.

I then repented for holding unforgiveness against those who had hurt me and openly forgave them again. Then my husband prayed for my deliverance from those spirits that had been tormenting me – because I had given them a place. God was faithful to His Word. He forgave me instantly, and I went to sleep in peace. When I awoke the next morning, there was absolutely no smell of garbage, and I have never been bothered with it again since that day. This example is relatively minor, but we can see from it that when we operate in unforgiveness, we leave ourselves open to evil spiritual forces that can affect our physical body negatively. It's just not worth it.

If you would stay healthy, refuse to hold grudges or resentments of any kind. Make it a practice to forgive others instantly and completely, and then ask God to help you to forget the sin as He does. If the enemy should try to remind you of a wrong you've forgiven, refuse to meditate on it and remind the devil that it is forgiven. You'll be surprised, after taking a firm stand like this for a while, just how hard you have to try to remember past sins against you; and you won't want to.

Remember, don't go by feelings. Forgiveness is a decision of the will, under the control of the Spirit of God. Some people have fed their bitterness and unforgiveness so long that they have come to the place where their minds have made up excellent excuses for refusing to forgive. But faith doesn't reside in, or flow out of, our minds. It flows from our hearts, and the born-again heart is created to love even the unlovable – because it is the heart of Jesus Himself. That's why it's important to remember that forgiving someone is a decision of the born-again spirit. It has nothing to do with feelings or emotions. Once we genuinely forgive, the emotions will eventually line up with that decision, but we can't wait for them to lead us because they are often controlled by our minds and will hold out against the heart if we give them the opportunity.

There's one more benefit to our walking in forgiveness, and that's the fact that our willingness to forgive and pray for those who have hurt us will often be the only avenue God has opened to Him to work on those individuals or to help them. God spoke a blessing onto Abraham when He made covenant with him, telling him that whoever blessed Abraham would be blessed, but whoever cursed Abraham would be cursed. You'll find the whole transaction recorded in Genesis 12:1-3.

Then God said that the promise was going to pass down to everyone of Abraham's descendants, and, in fact, He repeats the promise for the whole nation of Israel in Numbers 24:9. That means we, as believers, received that promise. Remember what we learned from Galatians, chapter 3: The curse of the law from the Old Covenant has been taken away by Jesus, so that we can receive the promises made to Abraham and all of his descendants – including everyone who becomes one with Jesus Christ.

Now, think about this point carefully. That promise means that if a person who is out of relationship with God does something to curse or harm you, he automatically opens himself up to harm. Now if he is a believer and recognizes his sin, he can certainly go to God and get it made right and give God an opportunity to intervene for him. But if he is not in relationship with God – or he refuses to repent and move into a position where the Lord can help him – then his only hope is if you decide to forgive that sin, ask the Lord to forgive him, and then pray for the Lord to intervene for him and help him. That's why Jesus, even when He was on the earth, taught people that there is a higher way to live than just by the law of the Old Covenant. He encouraged His followers, in the 5th chapter of Matthew, to not try to get even with those who hurt them, but to pray for them and bless them.

It would take far too many pages for me to relate the amazing results I've seen in real life when believers took the high road of forgiveness and blessing in response to those who had hurt them. Lives have been changed for eternity because of the open doors God had available to help those people, due to His own children following in the path of love and forgiveness.

So make a decision to put down your carnal nature that wants to retaliate or hold a grudge. Follow the calling of God's Spirit and make the decision to do what He does. Forgive. Just do it. The feelings will eventually follow. The best instructions I've found for how to forgive are recorded in the Amplified translation of Mark 11:25.

"And whenever you stand praying, if you have anything against anyone, forgive him and let it drop -- leave it; let it go ."

==============

Not Wanting To Be Well

Sometimes people do not receive healing because they really do not want to be completely well. There are certain people who feel the need for extra attention that comes with being sick. Family members will be willing to do things for them if they have continuing symptoms which make it difficult or impossible for them to function normally, and friends and family will ask about them often and allow them to discuss, at length, their various complaints.

Also, there are those people who do not want to take care of their rightful responsibilities at work or at home, and certain symptoms will allow them to leave those responsibilities for someone else without looking bad to others. I have even known people who actually enjoyed going to the doctor because that doctor gave them undivided attention while they were there. They were even delighted when they found out that they had certain illnesses and could be put on several kinds of medication.

Dear Christian, the book of James says that a double-minded man will receive nothing from the Lord. We must make up our minds that, if we want to be well, we must give up all of the self-serving, self-pitying attitudes and desires that come from being sick, and hunger with all our heart for real health that will make us able to be up and active and productive in this life. You know, even Jesus indicated this when He was ministering to the sick. In John 5:6, Jesus asked a man who had been sick for thirty-eight years, *"Do you wish to get well?"* We may be able to fool others, perhaps even ourselves, but, dear one, we will never fool the Beloved Physician. We must want health, along with its responsibilities, with all of our heart if we would have it from His hand.

============

Looking at Symptoms Instead of the Word

One of the most common hindrances to receiving healing from the Lord alone is our overwhelming human tendency to look at the physical symptoms rather than the Word of God. There are times, of course, when Christians pray for healing or are ministered to in a meeting of believers when the gifts of healings and miracles are in operation, and the manifestation of the healing comes instantly. However, when we are not in the presence of those gifts, there is still healing promised to us by the Lord. This healing comes as a result of our believing His Word, praying the prayer of faith for our healing, and praising Him for watching over His Word to perform It in our bodies and minds.

In the time period between praying for our healing and actually seeing it manifested, we will be severely tempted to look at any symptoms that remain in our bodies and question the reality of our healing. This time is the hardest test for any believer. Don't misunderstand; the idea is not to deny that symptoms exist or that a disease has developed in the body. Those things are real. The secret, however, lies in understanding that there is also a spiritual realm in which something else exists that's very real: healing. We must realize that healing and all other things in the spiritual realm are actually

more real than anything physical and can overcome and change anything in the natural, physical realm.

Some may ask, "Isn't this just mind over matter or wishful thinking?" No indeed! We are talking about reality here. Hebrews 11:1 says, *"Now faith is the substance of things hoped for, the evidence of things not seen."* Right away you can see that there are evidently some very **real** things in a realm where we cannot see them or perceive them with our five physical senses. We can add to this verse, 2 Corinthians 4:18, which says:

> *" ... while we look not at the things which are seen, but at the things which are not seen; for the things which are seen are temporal* (subject to change)*, but the things which are not seen are eternal."*

So things in the natural realm are temporary and changeable, but things – **real things** – in the spiritual realm are unchangeable and everlasting. Which realm is more powerful, dear Christian?

If there are any skeptics left, let's look at one more Scripture. Genesis 1:1 says, *"In the beginning God..."* There was nothing in the beginning except God – Who is a Spirit, according to the words of Jesus. *"In the beginning God created..."* When God decided to create the heavens and the earth, He had no raw materials to work with – only Himself, the Spirit God, and He created every single natural thing out of His own Spirit. Now, if spirit created matter, spirit has the power to change matter. That's why Jesus could say that if we have the faith of God, we can speak to a physical mountain, and it will obey us. The material mountain will obey the spirit of its Creator, when evidenced through that Creator's Word and faith.

So how do we develop faith in these unseen spiritual things and come into a place of receiving them manifested in the natural? By constantly looking at the one and only thing that shows us these spiritual realities: the Word of God. Romans 10:17 says, *"So faith comes from hearing, and hearing by the Word of God."* It is God's Word that makes us believe there **are** real spiritual things that are greater than those we can see. Wasn't it His Word that showed us there was a God in the first place and thereby created faith in us to believe in Him? Isn't it the Word that convinced us of Heaven and Hell? Of course. And that same Word is the only thing that will tell us of all the other spiritual realities, including healing.

2 Timothy 3:16 says, *"All Scripture is inspired by God ..."* That word **inspired** literally **means "God-breathed"**. That means that just as God breathed out the words, *"Let there be light,"* and they created light, so He has breathed out of Himself every word in the Bible, and these words created the very things He spoke. They still do creative work when **we** speak them in faith. As we devour that Word, It produces faith for those things that It shows us. That's why when we pray for something we can't see, we must make a decision to look only at the Word that verifies that thing we've asked for, and not give place to anything contrary shown us by our physical senses.

God, Who is Spirit, watches faithfully over His Word to perform It. He gives all spiritual things to us through our spirits. That's why we believe we receive **when we pray**. We **do** receive, by our spirit first. Our spirit lays hold of the gifts of God, and then, as faith is exercised, those gifts are brought into the natural.

Now healing is actually a spiritual thing that needs to be brought into the natural by faith. Just as God created light when He spoke the Word and called it forth, so He created healing for all mankind when He spoke the Word, as in Isaiah 53: 4-5, saying, *"... and by His scourging, we are healed."* We must recognize that the healing is a real thing, in the spirit realm, and that our faith applying the Word of God to our body, will draw that real healing into the natural and overpower the natural sickness, forcing it to change.

Sometimes this process takes a period of time. When Jesus cursed the fig tree in Mark, chapter 11, it did not manifest a change until the next day. However, I have no doubt that the curse went into effect on the roots of that tree immediately. It just took a while to show up on the branches. So with our bodies – the prayer of faith, and speaking the Word, puts God's power to work at the root of our sickness, and as we remain open to the work of that power by continuing to speak the Word and praise the Lord, it perfects its work in us. Sometimes, this takes a few hours; sometimes it can take as long as a year or so.

We don't always know why some work takes longer than others. Perhaps at times it's because we need more time to grow in the Word and better resist the enemy's temptation to give up and quit fighting the fight of faith. It is a fight sometimes, because the enemy wants us to believe that God doesn't mean what He says.

If he can keep our eyes on the symptoms long enough, we will doubt our Father's Word. Perhaps there are also times when the Lord, as a loving parent, wants us to grow up spiritually. He wants us to learn how to apply His Word in faith to our bodies and to stand on the truth of It. Learning that lesson, like learning any natural skill, takes a while.

Regardless of why the work takes time, we must decide to look only at our Lord and His faithfulness. We don't deny the symptoms. They are real. But they are real in the natural, remember, and the reality of healing from the spiritual realm is more real and more powerful. We just simply choose to lay hold of the healing and praise God for its reality until it does its work and overcomes the sickness.

The centurion in Matthew, chapter 8, told Jesus that all He had to do was speak the word, and his servant would be healed. We are told that when he returned home, he found that his servant had been healed in the same hour as Jesus had spoken. But the centurion had received the healing and started home without seeing the manifestation. The ten lepers in Luke 17 cried out to Jesus for healing. He told them to begin acting like they were healed and go to the priest, who was the one responsible for proclaiming them well according to their Jewish law. These ten men had no physical evidence of healing when they started off to find the priest. However, in the process of their acting on the Word of God, they received manifestation.

So we too must determine to obey the Word that says we are healed and act like it to the best of our ability. We must stand against fear when it comes; and it will surely come. For the enemy's best tool in defeating healing is causing us to fear that, for some reason, we will not receive our healing from God. Refuse to fear. Trust your God. Say only what His Word says about healing. We must also determine to have patience. Hebrews 10:35-36 says:

> *"Cast not away, therefore, your confidence, which hath great recompense of reward. For you have need of patience, that, after ye have done the will of God, ye might receive the promise."* (KJV).

There have been many instances in my own life when these words have proven true. I can remember several times when I had prayed the prayer of faith for my own healing, or had asked other believers to lay hands on me and pray for me, and received the healing by faith without seeing any instant change in symptoms. But as I stayed in the Word of God and gave Him my attention and praise, the symptoms totally disappeared without my having to turn to man's remedies.

Sometimes those battles of faith were mild, but a few times they were intense to the point of trying my faith to the limit. But thank God, when we come to the end of **our** faith, God meets us with His special gift of faith and carries us through. The great evangelist Smith Wigglesworth testified to this truth years ago: "Oh, this wonderful faith of Jesus Christ," he related. "Your faith comes to an end. How many times I have been to the place where I have had to tell the Lord, 'I have used all the faith I have,' and then He has placed His own faith

within me." (Smith Wigglesworth, *Ever Increasing Faith,* revised edition, Gospel Publishing House, p. 136.)

I experienced many nights of battle, sometimes devoting all night to listening to the Word on tape and speaking it to my situation. Sometimes I had to call on other believers to continue in prayer with me, holding onto God's faithfulness when there was nothing in the natural to hold on to. But God always came through, beloved, when I had made total commitment of myself to Him in every area.

You may have experienced the fact yourself that one of the most intense times of battle for spiritual things comes in the night or the wee hours of the morning. The enemy is a master at taking advantage of the darkness and the aloneness of the night hours to harass us unmercifully. But, beloved, the Word says that light and darkness are both alike to God, and He never leaves us nor forsakes us, so we will win, if we determine to remain faithful. And don't hesitate to call on other believers, if you are blessed with believing friends, because we are all in need of the strength of each other.

Some scoffers have made the point that they would not want to have to believe God for healing if it took that long and required that much work. Yet, they are willing to undergo medical treatment by human physicians that is painful, even agonizing, to their body. They will return time and time again for months, or even years, with only a **hope** that such treatment will stay the course of their disease. How much more do I prefer applying God's Word and prayer faithfully, even for months or years, having the **certainty** that His medicine will give me an absolute and complete cure every time.

I have had a couple of experiences in which I have prayed for healing but knew in my spirit that I did not have the peace that I had received it. I knew immediately what I had to do. I realized that I had not been faithfully in the Word for a period of time prior to the physical attack and that I had to shut out everything else for a day or two and devour the Word, especially the healing Scriptures. By the time I had **fed** on the Word for that length of time, **looking only at It**, my faith was ignited, and I knew without a doubt that I had the healing, even though symptoms hadn't changed yet. They did change, though; they had to! Yours will too!

====================

Failure to Submit to God in All Areas

There are times when we want something from the Lord, but we want it on our own terms. This problem can arise with healing. As we said earlier, all gifts that come to us from the Lord Himself are spiritually administered, and require an open channel from us to the Father in order to receive without hindrance. One of the most common ways of blocking this channel is disobedience on our part. God wants us to have all He has to give, but He has bound Himself by His Word to certain spiritual laws that govern His relationship with man, and they will not change. One of those laws is that when we submit ourselves completely to God, we come under His covenant protection, and He then fights our battles. That's why James 4:7 says, *"Submit therefore to God. Resist the devil and he will flee from you,"* Notice,

68

submission must come first; then, and only then, resisting the enemy will work. Once we are totally submitted to God, He stands tall behind us in every area of our lives, and the devil sees Him, and all of Heaven's power, coming at him when we resist him. However, if there are areas of our lives that we have failed to submit to the Lord, the enemy sees that too, and he believes God's Word enough to know that an area of rebellion (lack of submission) is an area that is open to attack.

Ephesians 4:7 exhorts us to *"give no place to the devil."* Psalm 107:20 says, *"Fools because of their rebellious way were afflicted. Their soul abhorred all kinds of food; and they drew near to the gates of death."* Sometimes it's actually deliberate sin that opens the door to attack. We need to remember that sin is any kind of disobedience to God's instructions – not just His commandments. Any time we deviate from God's way of doing things, we are asking for trouble.

We see more and more in our society that such things as sexual sins result in terrible effects upon the human body. We only has to look at AIDS to see that our Lord has our best interest in mind when He tells us how to live. But we need to be aware also that seemingly less important instructions from the Lord still carry out the same spiritual laws. When we act contrary to them, we are open to trouble. Even the instructions to be temperate in our eating and drinking are vital to us. If we do not let the Lord be God of our appetites, we open ourselves up to sickness and disease. We don't have to become fanatics about our diet, but we do need to recognize that the Lord's advice on anything is always for our best interest.

However, our problem could sometimes be that we are just plain lazy spiritually – not in the Word and prayer – not being sober and vigilant. Our Lord warns us in 1 Peter 5:8-9:

> *"Be of sober spirit, be on the alert. Your adversary, the devil, prowls about like a roaring lion, seeking someone to devour. But resist him firm in your faith ..."*

When we get lazy about the things that build up our faith, we let the enemy in the door with his attack against us. Sometimes our own words open the door to him, again because we have not been staying in God's Word and letting It rule our tongue. So it is important to remember that at the first hint of something out of God's will trying to find a place in our life, we must faithfully and firmly **resist**.

When we want the Lord's healing, we need to be sure that we are truly the Lord's in every area. Submit to Him; then resist the enemy, and he **will** flee.

If we are looking to God for healing, and we don't see anything manifesting after a period of time, we need to check up on ourselves and make sure that we really are surrendered to God on all points. Actually, I've personally found it a good idea to check up on my submission at the **first sign** of sickness. That way, if I have left any area open to the enemy, I can get it back under God's government immediately.

The Lord won't leave us in a state of confusion about our obedience to Him. If we truly want to know how we stand and are willing look to Him through the

Word and prayer, He will tell us clearly if we need to correct something, and He will tell us how. Generally, recognizing our disobedience, sincerely repenting of it, and submitting to the Lord at the time, is sufficient. You needn't worry that there is some area of disobedience in your life, and you can't figure out what it is. God's not playing games, and, if you really want to know, and are open to His channels of communication (His Word, prayer, and counsel from Godly leaders), He will tell you. He will never condemn you, beloved. Condemnation comes from your enemy. If you feel a general state of condemnation and can't figure out what you've done wrong, that is not from God. He brings only conviction, and that is far different. Conviction will lead us to specifically know the problem, to be grieved over it, to repent of it, and put it away.

==============

Possible Need for Deliverance

Sometimes physical illnesses have a specific demonic spirit or inherited curse at the root of the problem, causing the manifestation in the body. We know from Revelation, chapter 12, that when Satan was cast out of Heaven because of his rebellion, one-third of the angels, who had rebelled with him, were cast out also. Most Bible scholars agree that these angelic beings, who are created spirits, make up the host of demonic spirits, under Satan's leadership, who are constantly attacking and afflicting human beings on earth.

Both the Old and New Testaments show these beings trying to manifest their character and their limited power through human vessels on earth, sometimes causing those humans to act in evil ways, and sometimes just causing them to suffer in body and mind. Thank God, His Word makes it clear that these demonic beings have no ability to resist the omnipotent power and all-encompassing authority of Jesus Christ.

Many times when Jesus was ministering to a person who needed healing, He simply cast out a demonic spirit, and the person was instantly relieved of all physical problems. Note Matthew 9:32-33, which says:

> *"And as they were going out, behold, a dumb man, demon-possessed, was brought to Him. And after the demon was cast out, the dumb man spoke; and the multitudes marveled..."*

Again we see this type of ministry in Matthew 17:14-18:

> *"And when they came to the multitude, a man came up to Him, falling on his knees before Him, and saying 'Lord, have mercy on my son, for he is a lunatic, and is very ill; for he often falls into the fire, and often into the water. And I brought him to Your disciples, and they could not cure him ... And Jesus rebuked him (the demon), and the demon came out of him, and the boy was cured at once."*

Now let's turn to the book of Luke. In chapter 13, verses 10 and 16, Jesus healed a woman who was bowed over and could not hold herself erect. Verse 11 describes her:

> *"And behold there was a "woman who for eighteen years had had a sickness caused by a spirit; and she was bent double, and could not straighten up at all. And when Jesus saw her, He called her over and said to her, 'Woman, you are freed from your sickness.' And He laid His hands upon her, and immediately she was made erect again, and began glorifying God."*

Then Luke 4:40-41 shows us a group meeting in which Jesus dealt with all kinds of diseases, including those caused by demons:

> *"And while the sun was setting, all who had any sick with various diseases brought them to Him, and laying His hands on every one of them, He was healing them. And demons also were coming out of many, crying out and saying, 'You are the Son of God!' And rebuking them, He would not allow them to speak. ..."*

We see the need for this same kind of ministry in many cases today. Several years ago, the eldest son of some close friends was suffering with epilepsy. He went for prayer at his church, and as the pastor and other believers laid hands on him and prayed for his healing, one of those present saw a black form rise from his body and move through the air and out of the building. The young man was set free from all the symptoms of epilepsy at that time. Obviously, that spirit had been the root of the problem.

Another example of healing coming as the result of dealing with a demonic spirit concerns ministry for deafness. Some friends and I prayed with two different ladies who were deaf in one ear, and when we rebuked the spirit of deafness, they could hear. One lady, a businesswoman, was delighted that she could finally use the telephone with that ear.

I've noticed that certain diseases, especially those that develop organisms and cells that destroy healthy body tissues, and those that cause malfunctioning or crippling of parts of the mind or body, are often the work of a spirit of infirmity that has attached itself to the afflicted person. That's why a disease like cancer can be destroyed in one area of the body, with no sign of it showing up on tests, and then shows up again later in an entirely different part of the body. Sometimes that spirit of cancer has to be cast out. That's also why, many times, people with crippling arthritis have been set free instantly when the spirit of infirmity that had been binding up their limbs was cast out.

There is also a spirit of death that has attacked people, intending to end their life long before God is ready. It can be dealt with in the same way. Several years ago, while I was leading a home Bible study, a woman visiting the group for the first time began to look faint during praise and worship time. I had my eyes closed but was suddenly drawn to open my eyes and look directly at her.

As I did so, she began to slump in her chair, both arms falling limp to her sides. She had been speaking softly, but her words gradually drained away, and it seemed as though her breath did too. She turned a gray color, and I heard the Spirit of God speak in my own spirit that we were dealing with death. A nurse, who also attended the Bible study, was sitting across from this lady, and she was also led to open her eyes and look directly at her. Immediately recognizing the symptoms of death, she became very alarmed.

I knew the next move was up to me, but I seemed to be momentarily glued to my seat, praying in tongues. Everyone has had experiences in which a multitude of different thoughts flash through your mind all at once, and time seems to stand still while you think each one, although in reality everything takes place in split seconds. That was one of those experiences. In those split seconds, I was praying desperately for God to tell me what to do. I strained to hear His voice while simultaneously seeing newspaper headlines flash across my mind reading, "Woman Dies in Charismatic Bible Study".

Then I suddenly felt as if a spring had been released on the seat of my chair, and I popped up, stepped over to that woman, laid hands on her head, and commanded the spirit of death to leave her. The others were praying fervently, both in English and in tongues. I then commanded life to come into every part of her and prayed for healing as well.

When I spoke the command for life to come into her, she began to breath noticeably again, color came back into her flesh, and within seconds she came back to consciousness. In a few minutes, she was able to sit up and carry on with the class.

She shared with us later that some weeks earlier, an individual "claiming" to have knowledge from the Lord, had told her she would die an early death. She had accepted that, received the spirit of death, and succumbed to it. After that meeting, that little lady was so alive and so excited to know God wanted her to be that way, that she was a joy to be around and a real blessing to that Bible study.

Another interesting note to this testimony, which shows how God works behind the scenes to take care of us, concerns my husband. At the time of this meeting, he was at home, about forty miles away, when, all of a sudden, he sensed the Holy Spirit speak in his heart these words: "A woman is going to die in Sandy's Bible study today." He looked at the clock, noting that the Bible study had started, and immediately began to pray for God to intervene. I'll always believe that his prayers were mainly responsible for my finally being able to spring from my chair and take authority over that spirit of death in Jesus' name. How good God is. When we walk with Him, He works in a multitude of ways to deliver and protect us.

========================

Curses

There are also times when a physical disease is the result of a curse for sin on the lives of previous generations, which has been carried down to us genetically and never dealt with by the power of the blood of Jesus. When God cursed sin, that curse, like all of the rest of God's Word, was settled forever in heaven. God does not change, and that means His promises **and** His curses are still in effect in the earth. The glorious truth for us, however, is that mercy has triumphed over judgment, and the suffering of Jesus wrought the power to break the curse legally and set us free from it. But we must know the truth and how to walk in it.

It is not the purpose of this book to do a thorough study of genetic curses. However, I will cite a few verses that will establish the fact that they do exist and that Jesus is the way to overcome them. First of all, let's look at Deuteronomy, chapter 28. As previously noted, this chapter of Deuteronomy gives us the clear and concise statement of God, concerning the results of our obedience and disobedience to His commandments. The first fourteen verses deal with the wondrous blessings on obedience. But beginning with verse 15, we can see the horrendous results of disobedience. Let us look specifically at verses 15 and 18:

> *"But it shall come about, if you will not obey the Lord your God, to observe to do all His commandments and His statutes with which I charge you today, that all these curses shall come upon you and*

*overtake you. Cursed shall be the offspring
of your body..."*

Then, let us look at Exodus 20:4-6:

*"You shall not make for yourself an idol,
or any likeness of what is in heaven above
or on the earth beneath or in the water
under the earth. You shall not worship
them or serve them; for I the Lord your
God am a jealous God, visiting the iniquity
of the fathers on the children, on the third
and the fourth generations of those who
hate Me, but showing loving-kindness to
thousands, to those who love Me and keep
My commandments."*

Even in the earthly ministry of Jesus, we see that this
spiritual law was still in operation, according to Matthew
23:19-33. Jesus says:

*"Woe to you scribes and Pharisees,
hypocrites! For you build the tombs of the
prophets and adorn the monuments of the
righteous, and say, 'If we had been living
in the days of our fathers, we would not
have been partners with them in shedding
the blood of the prophets.' Consequently,
you bear witness against yourselves, that
you are sons of those who murdered the
prophets. Fill up then the measure of the
guilt of your fathers. You serpents, you*

brood of vipers, how shall you escape the sentence of hell?"

According to the record of this conversation in Luke 11:47-51, Jesus then adds the following:

"For this reason also the wisdom of God said, 'I will send to them prophets and apostles, and some of them they will kill and some they will persecute, in order that the blood of all the prophets, shed since the foundation of the world, may be charged against this generation, from the blood of Abel to the blood of Zechariah, who perished between the altar and the house of God; yes I tell you, it shall be charged against this generation.'"

You see, many times, not only does the curse pass down, but even the same weaknesses and tendencies to certain kinds of sin are carried from generation to generation. But, beloved, remember that Galatians 3:13 says: *"Christ has redeemed us from the curse of the law, being made a curse for us..."*

We must apply this truth and the blood of Jesus to our situation to break the power of these genetic curses and inclinations of the flesh, just as we apply the blood and the Word to any sickness to destroy its power over us.

Many may ask, "But can a Christian have a demon or be under a curse?" It is important to note here that a Christian is one who is born again of the Spirit of God

Himself and has been made a new and righteous creature in his spirit-man. Therefore, no demon can **possess** a Christian because it cannot take up residence in the spirit, the inner man, in which Jesus reigns. However, a demon **can attach itself** to a Christian, just as disease germs can, particularly when we don't know our legal rights in Christ to be free from these things. You see, we have to apply the sacrifice of our Lamb, Jesus, and the Word – which is the power of God – and resist the devil, whether in the form of a demon, a disease, or a sin.

We must also realize that disobedience to God opens us up to this kind of attack by the enemy. He will take all the ground we let him have, whether by our ignorance or our disobedience. In the same way, curses can operate in our lives, even though we are Christians, either because we don't know the Word well enough to recognize them as curses that we can break; or because we have entered into some sin that brings them into operation.

It is a sad fact that babies are often born into this world carrying the physical effects of those genetic curses. A thorough study of God's Word will bring to light a direct connection between some specific kinds of sins and specific diseases or impairments. "But it's not the baby's fault," you may say. "Why should he suffer?" We must remember that every human being born into this world has suffered, in one way or another, as the result of the sin of our original parents. As Romans 5:12-14 says:

> *"Therefore, just as through one man sin entered into the world, and death through sin, and so death spread to all men,*

because all sinned – for until the Law sin was in the world; but sin is not imputed when there is no law. Nevertheless death reigned from Adam until Moses, even over those who had not sinned in the likeness of Adam's offense, who is a type of Him who was to come."

But then the Lord says in verses 15-19:

"But the free gift is not like the transgression. For if by the transgression of one the many died, much more did the grace of God and the gift by the grace of the one Man, Jesus Christ, abound to the many . . . For if by the transgression of the one, death reigned through the one, much more those who receive the abundance of grace and of the gift of righteousness will reign in life through the One, Jesus Christ. So then as through one transgression there resulted condemnation to all men, even so through one act of righteousness there resulted justification of life to all men. For as through the one man's disobedience the many were made sinners, even so through the obedience of the One the many will be made righteous."

Knowing these truths, we can see that it is so very important that Christian parents pray for their children from the time of conception and speak the living Word of God to that child even in the womb. By the authority of

Jesus, they can break the power of any disease or addiction that has been active in the bloodline of either side of the family. Also, they should bind the devil from imposing any tendency to specific sins that are known to have plagued the family. The parents have this God-given authority, assuming, of course, that they are walking in obedience and right relationship to the Lord themselves. Parents involved in unclean or ungodly habits or lifestyles automatically open the door for demonic attack on their children.

We see another common example of inherited curses in many alcoholics. We know that everyone who drinks intoxicating beverages doesn't necessarily become an alcoholic. There is something specific taking place in the ones who do. Many times these people have parents, grandparents, or great-grandparents who were alcoholics. They have inherited the weaknesses that make them unable to tolerate alcohol in a controlled form, and they also inherit that spirit of addiction that drives them to drink it incessantly. You see, that spirit of addiction is allowed to come in through the sin of an ancestor; and its resulting curse. (A curse provides the conditions for a demonic spirit to operate legally.)

This fact explains why sometimes people can become Christians but find they still have a serious problem with alcohol. They need to apply the name and the blood of Jesus to break the effects of those sins that originally brought the curse into operation and to cast that spirit out. Jesus paid the price for the deliverance, but we often need to apply the power of His finished work by faith for its manifestation, just as we need to apply that power for healing of a broken bone or a sore throat.

Another area where we see people commonly suffering as a result of inherited curses, and spirits of infirmity, is the disease of cancer. To be sure, many times our lifestyle and the way we eat open us up to deviations in the development of cells, but even medical science recognizes today that the tendency to develop cancer is definitely carried genetically for generations. But here again, it's knowing that Jesus set us free **legally** and applying the Word of truth in faith to whatever is attacking us that sets us free **experientially**.

And how do we apply that Word and that power? By believing it and acting and speaking as if we believe it. Why is **speaking** so important in these situations? Remember, God said in Proverbs, *"Life and death are in the power of the tongue."* Jesus said that whatever is in a man's heart, he will speak out of his mouth, and the book of James says that faith without works is dead. Now that word **works** in the original Greek means "corresponding action". So our action and words will show forth our faith if it is alive. Then we have the words of authority that Jesus gave to the church in Matthew 18:18:

> *"Truly I say to you, whatever ye shall bind on earth shall be bound in heaven and whatever you loose on earth shall be loosed in heaven."*

You see, God created by His Word. He established His whole relationship with us by His Word, and when Jesus came to earth in the flesh, He operated the power of

God primarily through His words. Words release power. So it's important for us to speak God's words, in order for His power to be released to overcome the enemy in our life.

Now I trust that discussion of this particular hindrance does not produce fear in any reader who has come to this book for help. Remember, beloved, fear is not from our Lord. Nor should you allow yourself to feel condemned if you feel that you are suffering from a physical problem that is caused by a demonic spirit or an inherited curse. Many times the person suffering has not been guilty of any of the specific sins that originally opened the door to this demonic attack. The demonic power has simply become operational in that person's life or his body through his natural bloodline. It must be recognized for what it is and gotten rid of by the power of Jesus.

This particular hindrance is simply **one** of the areas of spiritual battle connected with sickness. If you have been suffering from a physical problem, and general prayer in faith has not brought the desired manifestation, it is time to ask the Lord if there is some specific hindrance involved in the delay of the physical results you seek. If you are asking from an honest and sincere heart and are giving God every opportunity to reveal Himself to you – by being in His Word, in prayer, and in consistent fellowship with other believers – He will always show you what the hindrance is and how to deal with it effectively. Remember that removing any hindrance to a miracle is as easy as any other work that we need the Lord to do for us, as long as we are willing to do our part obediently.

The very Word of God Itself has the power to drive out evil spirits. If we will saturate ourselves with that Word and speak It to our situation, It will do the work. But many times people need immediate help even before they can saturate themselves with the Word. Because of that, I would like to make special note here that in dealing with this particular type of hindrance, it is a great advantage to be in a committed relationship with a body of believers overseen by a pastor and elders.

Through the gifts of the Holy Spirit, operating in other believers, and the anointing on the offices of leadership, the Lord can very easily and quickly reveal and destroy the hold of demons and genetic curses. Beloved, when the Lord told us to be diligent to join ourselves together regularly with other believers, He did so because He knew we all need each other's help.

(Special Anointing on Leadership)

It might be good to say an extra word here about the spiritual authority inherent in the offices of a God-called pastor or elder. I am not referring to those men or women who take on those offices as a result of self-desire; or the desire of other men. But when God calls a man into the office of pastor or elder, and he accepts it faithfully, that man walks into a position of extraordinary power in the spiritual realm. Why? Because God has ordained that these positions of leadership carry the weight of the spiritual development and protection of the body over which they are shepherds. In order for them to be able to fulfill this responsibility, God has allotted to the office itself a particular degree of spiritual dominion, recognized by all of heaven and feared by all of hell.

When the pastor speaks and acts in the duties of his office, heaven's forces and hell's forces stand at attention, ready to respond: The former to bless, and the latter to flee. It never ceases to thrill me when I contemplate this truth. It shows me God's unwavering faithfulness to His Word. He has set this divine government of His people into operation, and He will see to it that it works effectively for the good of His kingdom.

Now that does not mean that God will not answer the simplest believer's prayer just as surely and as quickly as He will the pastor's. As a matter of fact, it is a very sad truth that, even though the authority resides in the office, if a pastor or elder has not fed on the Word of God and spent time in prayer until that Word becomes alive in him, he will not have the faith to operate in that God-ordained authority. All of the dominion that is resident in his office lies dormant for want of a living faith in God's Word. But let that man believe God, and there's no holding back what God can do.

God responds faithfully to love and faith in operation anywhere and everywhere He finds them – in the newest Christian or the oldest pastor. But in the midst of intense spiritual conflict over a problem we are facing, it is good to know that one of our spiritual weapons is the anointing that comes with the office of authority and to make use of it when really necessary.

I have done this personally on a few different occasions in my life. I recall two different times, about three years apart, that I was having a battle with severe pain and pressure in my head. The problems were not connected, as the cause was different in each case. My husband and I prayed in agreement for the deliverance I needed. I spent much time in the Word and would get temporary relief, but nothing permanent.

During the first experience, I told my husband (after about three days) that I felt I should have our pastor pray for me, because there kept rising up in my spirit the reminder that there is specific spiritual authority in his office that could break the power of that physical problem. So my husband and I stopped by our pastor's house, and when he prayed, I felt relief instantly and had complete deliverance by the next day.

On the second occasion, a Resurrection Sunday morning, I arose from a totally sleepless night, having suffered for four days with the most agonizing symptoms, in spite of our persistence in prayer and the Word. I knew in my heart that God had heard and given the answer. Yet, I had been under siege by the enemy and his unceasing symptoms and lies all night. I knew I had to have more of God's army on the battlefront. Shortly after I got up, I recalled that several of the church leaders would be meeting early that morning for prayer before service, and I felt a leading to call and ask them to pray for me.

When my pastor answered the phone, he said they would be glad to pray for me, but then he said, "Let me pray for you right now." He proceeded to take authority in the name of Jesus over that thing that had tormented me for days. I immediately knew in my spirit that he was sure of his authority as my pastor, and that he was also sure of the finished work of Christ. The consciousness of the full victory of the resurrection rang in his voice. From the second the words were out of his mouth, I felt the power that had bound me for days break completely and loose my head. The pain, the pressure, and the dizziness left, and I was free.

Now I do not relate this truth to imply that any time a Christian is sick he should run to his pastor. On the contrary, we need to learn to believe God for ourselves. However, knowing that we are in a spiritual warfare, and knowing that the Lord has given us a complete arsenal of spiritual weapons to use, we do not want to be ignorant of which weapon is the best one for each particular attack. We must know the **whole** counsel of God and walk in it if we would have constant victory.

=============

Lack of Ministry from the Local Body

The last hindrance we will discuss does not reside in the one seeking healing. Rather, it resides in the Body of Christ in general, and more so in some parts of the Body than others. The average body of believers in our day does not really believe the Word of God 100 percent. We want to think that we do. We are sometimes offended if anyone implies that we do not believe completely. But the sad fact is that Jesus could have been looking down the centuries and speaking to *us* when He said, *"Oh, unbelieving generation...."*

Most of the adult Christians in the world today have been reared in a society that has had its gospel so subtly watered down by false teachings and the doctrines of men that we have never learned to take God's Word for what It says and structure every particle of our lives by It. Oh, we've been taught that God loves us and sent Jesus to save us from our sins. We've been taught the stories of God's miraculous intervention into all areas of men's lives in the pages of Scripture, but too often we see them as just pretty little stories or parables to teach us something about what God used to do – but not something that we can expect in our own lives in every situation. We have been reared in churches that have compromised their faith because they have believed for so long that they had to use man's ways and means to accomplish anything in the natural.

I recognize this sad truth in so many areas of life, but we must deal primarily here with the area of healing. It has been my experience that a Christian can rarely ask other church members, even in Full Gospel churches, for prayer for physical problems that seems serious without receiving responses such as, "Well, have you gone to the doctor?" or, "What did the doctor say about it?" or, "You had better see a doctor about that. It could be really serious." And then I can't count the number of times I've heard, "You know you don't want to be a fanatic. After all, God expects us to use doctors."

As we said in the first chapter, Jesus, Who is the exact representation of God's will on the earth, never ever suggested to one seeking healing that he should seek out a human doctor, even though doctors were in common practice at the time. And if we look at the church in the book of Acts, and any other credible history of the early church for about the first 300 years, we find that believers didn't even consider that option for receiving healing. They did what the Lord Himself instructed them to do according to Mark 16 and James 5. They laid hands on the sick and expected them to be healed, and they called the elders, anointed with oil, and prayed prayers of faith. Of course, they also stayed in the Word, stayed in fellowship, and fasted and prayed often, so they were not overcome by unbelief. Today, we Christians live so much in the world, concentrating on the way the world thinks and how the world's leaders suggest we handle problems that we aren't in the Word enough. We don't fast and pray often. We don't spend every possible moment available to us in the presence of Almighty God, so we don't stay filled with the Spirit and the Word, ready to believe with a brother or sister, or to minister to their need.

Another side of the same coin is that we often have a few believers who will pray with a brother or sister about a physical problem for a period of time, but if the manifestation does not come, or symptoms become critical, they back off and say something like, "Well, Brother, if you are not able to believe for a miracle yourself, you had better go ahead and have an operation, or you might die." Dear Christian, do you see that that is not the way of the Word? God says, if one is sick, he should not have to believe for himself; rather, there should be those mature in the faith that will anoint with oil, pray the prayer of faith, and do the believing for the sick one.

One particular experience with a problem like this comes to my mind so clearly at this time. Several years ago, there was a sister who went to church where my husband and I attended, who had been experiencing some severe symptoms in her female organs. She had sought prayer from some sisters in the faith and had been ministered to more than once in a Bible study group. A doctor had examined her and told her she needed to have a complete hysterectomy, as well as possible surgery for her bladder. When she did not show any improvement in the symptoms after a period of time, the sisters who had prayed for her told her that if she were not able to believe for a miracle for herself, she should go and have the surgery, citing another person who had been prayed for and died.

When she related this experience to me a short time after the other women had given up on her, I just felt indignant at the way the devil has deceived God's people. The glorious compassion of God rose up in me so strongly, and I said, "Sister, that's just not so." I explained to her that God had made provision for the body of believers to carry the sick one who was not able to do all the believing for himself. I explained that it was the body's responsibility to work its faith on her behalf. New faith was ignited in her heart, and new light came into her eyes at this news.

We went to work rounding up some of the elders of the body and explained the situation, telling them that she needed others to fight the fight of faith **for** her – and so we did. A couple of weeks later, that sister was feeling better, and she decided to go to see another doctor and see what he had to say about her condition. When he examined her, he told her that there was no need for surgery of any kind. Before long, every negative symptom was gone, and that sister believed God to cause her and her husband to have another child.

Beloved, we can't keep looking back at the Old Testament patriarchs, or the apostles of the early church, and saying, "It's too bad they are not living today so that they could believe like that for us or perform the same miracles today." We can't look back to the turn of the century, when there were a hand-full of ministers full of the Holy Spirit who brought miraculous healing to hundreds of thousands in meetings all over the world, and say, "It's a shame we don't have more people like that today." No, beloved Christian! It's time we faced facts. We – WE – You and I – are the giants of faith for today. You may say, "Boy, are we a pitiful excuse for giants!" AMEN! We are – but we don't have to be. Let's recognize that God is still the same God, and He'll still do the same glorious things if He can just find people who will spend enough time with Him to be able to **really believe Him without reservation and without qualification.**

The Lord's looking for those unselfish enough to get into the fight with one who needs a miracle of healing from God and determine to **stay** in the fight until the victory comes. Sometimes that will mean praying around the clock with the sick one for several days at a time. Sometimes, it will mean praying every day with that one for months. Other times, it will mean being willing to fast and pray until the Spirit of discernment shows the hindrance; or the gifts of healings and miracles come into operation. Sometimes, it will mean reading the healing Scriptures to the sick one day after day after day, until they're strong enough to get hold of them for themselves. Instead of saying, "Give up and go to the doctor", we need to say, "Hang on; God's fighting for you, and so am

I. You'll get the victory." But we need to say it, not because it sounds good, but because we believe it --because we **know** it -- because we're so full of God Himself.

Now, Dear Christian, if you're sick, you have the right to believe for your own healing all by yourself. But if you're having trouble alone, don't waste your time hanging around people who don't believe God. Find as many people as you possibly can who really believe what the Word says about healing and spend as much time with them as you can. Then, after you're healed, keep spending time with them.

It's amazing how many people have experienced a miraculous healing from the Lord, only to be talked out of it by people in their own family or their own church. I'll never forget a young girl who came to the church I attended many years ago. She had one leg shorter than the other, and when she was prayed for, she received a miracle. Her short leg was made normal by the power of God and became the same length as the other one. She was able to feel, as well as see, the work being done on her leg by the Lord. Needless to say, she was excited.

But when she went back to her home church, where they did not believe that God still performs healing miracles today the way that He did while on earth in the flesh, they convinced that poor girl that what she had received wasn't real at all. As she listened to their continual browbeating, she began to believe them rather than the Lord -- and even her own experience. Her leg responded to the unbelief in her heart and mouth, and it drew up again, shorter than the other one. When she realized what had happened, she returned to our church and was ministered to again. This time, it took much longer for her to receive the miracle, because of the tremendous stronghold of unbelief that had been established in her heart and mind.

But our great God is so merciful, and through the faith of the believers who gathered around her and prayed fervently, He was able to work His way through her unbelief and give her her miracle the second time. Dear One, if you want miracles from the Lord, guard yourself against those who would discourage you from believing.

And finally, beloved, determine in your heart to learn everything you can about God's healing, so that you will be full of the truth. Get filled with the Holy Spirit and stay in prayer and in the presence of God, so that you can stay filled. Be ready to help a brother or sister who needs healing. Don't be one who sends them away sorrowing, to the world's methods and failures. Believe God's Word and be a giant of faith for someone else!

Questions for Review:

1. According to the text, when someone is prayed for and does not receive healing, could the problem be that God didn't want to heal them?

2. Although we can get healed on someone else's faith, if we want to be sure of healing every single time in our own life, what must we study thoroughly?

3. Can there be healing without forgiveness of sins?

4. What is the only thing that will keep us from receiving God's forgiveness for our own sins?

5. Can unforgiveness affect us physically?

6. Is forgiveness a feeling or a decision?

7. List two reasons why some people prefer to be sick.

8. When we insist on saying what God's Word says instead of what our symptoms of illness say, are we denying the symptoms?

9. What is the only thing that can create faith?

10. Which realm is more real -- the spiritual or the natural?

11. According to James 4:7, to get the devil to flee from us, what must we do?

12. Name two things that can cause physical illness that people may need deliverance from.

13. Did Jesus ever indicate that a demon was responsible for someone's illness? Give two Scriptures to support your answer.

14. Can demonic assignments and curses be passed down to the next generation?

15. In order to apply God's delivering power to our own life or the lives of our loved ones, is it really important to speak His Word aloud?

16. Is there always deliverance available for demonic oppression or curses?

17. If a Christian does not have strong enough faith to believe all by himself for his healing from God, does that mean he should automatically give up and do whatever medical science says? Why?

18. Who is God counting on to be the giants of faith in the world today?

Questions for Meditation and Discussion:

1. When our circumstances or past experiences seem to be the opposite of what we see in the life of Jesus or in God's Word, what conclusion should we come to? What actions should we be moved to take to clear up such confusion?

2. How does unforgiveness keep us from receiving from God?

3. What is the difference between the "mind over matter" philosophy and standing in faith to receive something that we cannot yet see in the natural?

4. Is complete submission to God necessary if we want His blessings in our life? Why?

5. How is it that demonic spirits and curses can oppress a Christian? How can we be sure we walk free of these evils?

6. Why is it absolutely imperative for a Christian to be in a committed relationship with a body of believers?

7. Is it each Christian's responsibility to believe for his healing all by himself? What do you see as your own responsibility in helping the Body of Christ to be healed and to stay well?

MEANS OF HEALING PRESCRIBED
IN THE WORD

As we said in Chapter One, so far as we can find evidence from God's written Word, He has only one remedy for all sickness, whether of spirit, soul, or body – Jesus Christ. He alone broke the power of the curse that has resulted from sin.

However, perhaps we should take the opportunity here to state once more that God does not hold it against us if we are in a position where we believe we need to incorporate man's medical healing, along with the Lord. If you are a parent whose child is seriously ill, and you know that fear is making a stronger impression on you than the Scriptures you've read, you feel the need to call a human physician to get immediate relief for your child. You are perfectly free in God's sight to do so.

Or if you're suffering with a pounding headache, and your schedule is so tight that there's no time to sit down and listen to the Word on tape and meditate on it until it saturates your body; or perhaps your Word time hasn't been exactly up to par lately either, you can take two aspirin and go on your way without condemnation. God doesn't have us backed into a corner with a commandment that says, "Thou shalt never make use of human medical help."

However, He does know that human medical help is limited at best, and sometimes dangerous at its worst. He wants to draw us constantly up to believing for His own means of restoring our bodies to health. Our Lord has prescribed, in His Word, several means of getting the power of Jesus Christ into our bodies or souls to accomplish that healing. Different means are more effective for particular people at particular times. Since people are different and needs constantly change, the Lord, in His wisdom and love, has provided a full gamut of possibilities to make receiving from Him as easy as possible. Each believer will need to seek the Lord as to the avenue most effective for him at each given time. There may be times when several of these means will need to be applied at the same time.

We will look now at nine of the most common means the Lord uses to bring His healing to His children.

The Gifts of Healings and the Gift of Working of Miracles

The first means of healing we will consider is also the only one of the nine that is not available on a continuous basis and, therefore, not solely a matter of the believer's choice. This avenue of healing includes the gifts of healings (the word is plural in the original Greek) and the gift of working of miracles, described in 1 Corinthians 12:4-11.

"Now there are varieties of gifts, but the same Spirit, and there are varieties of ministries, and the same Lord. ... But to each one is given the manifestation of the Spirit for the common good. For to one is given the word of wisdom through the Spirit, and to another the word of knowledge ... and to another gifts of healing ... and to another the effecting of miracles .... But one and the same Spirit works all these things, distributing to each one individually just as He wills."

The nine ministry gifts listed in this passage are specific, supernatural manifestations of the Holy Spirit, which He activates at His will. Anyone who has been baptized in the Holy Spirit has the potential for being used for the operation of these gifts, but none of those individuals can operate the gifts at his personal discretion.

The gifts of healings and the gift of working of miracles often manifest through ministers in large group meetings, where corporate faith releases the power of God to flow especially freely. Often even unbelievers receive miracles of healing in such meetings because the hindrances are broken down by the massive release of faith of the body as a whole. Sometimes these same gifts operate in one-on-one ministry as well, but we find them most active in evangelistic meetings as an aid to convincing the masses of God's mercy and love.

The other distinctive characteristic of these gifts is that they are often in operation for specific health problems at specific times – not for general healing of any and every malady. As a result of the uniqueness of these particular gifts, there are often Christians who attend meetings where these gifts are in operation, but they do not receive the healing they needed personally. When that happens, it's encouraging to know that there are plenty more avenues to receive from the Lord that are not so restrictive.

All of the ***other means*** of healing discussed in this chapter differ from these gifts, in that every other means provided by the Lord is available on a continuous basis and can be accessed at any hour and for as long as necessary by every single believer. All of these remaining avenues of healing are also unrestricted and non-specific when it comes to the kinds of health problems they will relieve. They can be applied to absolutely any and every problem of body or soul.

Our Own Prayer of Faith

Jesus said in John 14:13-14, *"And whatever you ask in My name, that will I do, that the Father may be glorified in the Son. If you ask Me anything in my name, I will do it."* He also said in John 15:7, *"If you abide in Me, and My words abide in you, ask whatever you wish, and it shall be done for you."*

That word **abide** means **"to dig down deep, plant roots, and live there."** We need to dig deep into God's

101

Word, find out what He promised and what He requires, and live in that knowledge. Then we will have the faith to ask for what we need from Him.

We have looked at several individuals already who made their own request of faith to Jesus for healing: the leper, the Samaritan mother, the Roman centurion who told Jesus He needed only to speak the word to accomplish healing. And the gospels are full of others: the blind, the mute, the lunatics, the relatives of dying loved ones.

All these people asked Jesus for themselves, based on their own faith, which had grown from what they had learned of Him. And **not one** of them was denied. Each one received the healing he required of the Lord. If we look at the various stories carefully, we see that they all had two specific things in common: They had heard the good news that Jesus healed and believed it, and they all came worshiping Him or honoring Him as the anointed of God before they received their miracle. We must acknowledge Him as who He really is – the only true Savior and Lord; the only One with healing and life in His very nature.

When the Word tells us that Jesus was unable to do many great miracles in His hometown, it was not because the people believed in Him but were weak in their faith. No, it was because they **refused** to believe and accept Him as who He said He was. They were so unwilling to accept Him as the Messiah that they pushed Him to the edge of a hill and planned to throw Him off and kill Him. Beloved, it is not weak faith that keeps God from acting, but deliberate unbelief and refusal to submit to Him. Now weak faith may make things take a little longer, but as we stay in the Word, our faith will grow; and so will our ability to receive from God.

Remember that Mark 11:24 says: *"Therefore, I say to you, all things for which you pray and ask, believe that you have received them, and they shall be granted you."*

Philippians 4:6 says: *"Be anxious for nothing, but in everything by prayer and supplication with thanksgiving let your requests be made known to God."*

And 1 John 5:14-15 says: *"And this is the confidence which we have before Him, that if we ask anything according to His will, He hears us. And if we know that He hears us in whatever we ask, we know that we have the requests which we have asked from Him."*

Dear sick one, get hold of the promise; make your request on the basis of it; know that God grants it to you; and begin the process of praise, whereby the channels are kept fully open. And don't be discouraged if you feel the need to pray again. You don't have to ask the Lord repeatedly to grant the healing, because He does that as soon as you ask, but you may have to fight the battle of resisting symptoms, spiritual attacks, and the bad advice of other people; and the Lord wants you to run to Him for comfort and encouragement in believing until the answer is manifested.

I recall a time when my husband Richard had a blockage in the circulatory system of his foot. The foot swelled to twice its normal size and became red and ugly. We prayed and asked others to pray, and we then began to praise the Lord for the healing. The symptoms persisted for two weeks. Each time we looked at the foot, and fear tried to grip us, we reminded ourselves of what God's Word says.

Finally into the third week, due to a death in the family and the exhausting duties involved with that, we found ourselves totally exhausted one evening, both physically and spiritually, and still dealing with that swollen, ugly foot. The strain of everything together had me to the point of giving up, and fear was trying to get a foothold once again. I slumped into a chair, too tired and discouraged to pray out loud or even call someone else to pray for us. I cried out in my spirit, "Please, Lord, call on someone to pray for us right now. We're just too weak to go on."

Within the hour, our telephone rang. My husband answered, and it was a representative from the 700 Club in Virginia Beach, Virginia. Now they had called him from time to time in the past, explained a program they were working on for the Lord, and always asked for an offering to support them in the work. Before hanging up, they always offered to pray for any needs. However, this time the representative did not mention any program in the works or the need for any offering. He just asked immediately if Richard had any needs for prayer. Richard told him about his foot, and the brother prayed the prayer of faith for him and hung up. I felt as if a bolt of lightning had struck my heart. I can't tell you in words how my faith soared; just to think that God would move so supernaturally just to encourage us to believe.

We went to bed in perfect peace, confident of God's healing, and when we awoke the next morning, Richard's foot was normal size and normal color.

God had been holding out that healing to us in answer to all the previous prayers, but we were having a hard time receiving. When I turned to Him for help, He moved miraculously, tapping a man in Virginia on the shoulder and telling him to call long distance to pray for Richard as a sign to us that He really was working for us. He knew that particular act would quicken our faith and put us in a position to receive. He won't allow us to become spiritual weaklings, but when He knows we really need help, He never fails to give it.

Prayer of Agreement

In connection with our prayer of faith, we see that God has made provision for two or more believers to unite together for the same request. Perhaps you don't feel that you are prepared to stand in faith alone. Find another who knows the Word of God and knows how to use it in prayer, and agree with them in your request from the Father. Jesus told us in Matthew 18:19:

> *"Again I say to you, that if two of you agree on earth about anything that they make ask, it shall be done for them by My Father who is in heaven."*

What a promise! This promise is a particular blessing for believing husbands and wives. Many a victory has been won by the earnest, believing prayers of a husband and wife in perfect agreement.

I might add a word here also about the power in the prayers of the husband and father of a family. I can't help but chuckle as I think back to my first experiences with my husband's prayers for me. My husband has always been a man of few words. (I, on the other hand, have always been a woman of many.) During the first years of our marriage, when I needed prayer, my husband was always so faithful to take my need to the Lord. In his typical fashion, he spoke to the Lord very briefly and considered it done. I was frustrated, even a little aggravated, that he had made such short work of it – until I realized God had met my need in a very short time. My husband's short prayers and matter-of-fact faith usually got faster results for me than my long prayers did for him.

Because God Himself has designated the man as the head of the wife and family, high priest of the home if you will, He honors the sincere prayers of that man on behalf of his loved ones. Even men who may be far from being giants of faith find God faithful to honor the office in which the husband and father stands when he intercedes for his family. Divinely assigned spiritual authority carries with it Divinely endued spiritual power. As husbands and fathers, even those weak in faith, submit to God and accept their position as priests of the home, tremendous miracles take place for the whole family.

Laying on of Hands

Mark 16:18 says that believers will lay hands on the sick, and they will be healed. This practice was one of the means that Jesus used while on earth in the flesh because it provided a way to release the actual power of God into a person's flesh. The Spirit of God is a real person, and His power is the very energy that created the universe. It too is very real. Scientists and lab technicians have at times tested this power in laboratories with x-ray machines and machines that register energy flow. They have been able to show clinically that at the time of prayer, a real transfer of an energy force takes place and changes the flesh into which it flows. So when believers, filled with the same Holy Spirit that Jesus was filled with, lay hands on the sick in His name, that same power flows into and heals the sick.

Sometimes, when the healing is taking place gradually, and believers have laid hands on the sick one a number of times over a period of weeks, medical tests have shown definite physical improvement after each episode of prayer. We see an example of this in Scripture. When Jesus ministered to the blind man in Mark 8:22-25, He found that the man received part of his healing manifested the first time hands were laid on him, but received the complete manifestation after Jesus laid His hands on him a second time.

There is also another advantage in the laying on of hands. When one is sick, faced with very physical symptoms, the physical experience of feeling the believers' hands on his body allows the sick one to release his faith at the exact time of prayer, and often makes receiving easier. The Lord thinks of everything, beloved, and He know there are times that we need a particular kind of experience to help us receive from Him. It is probably for this reason also, that the laying on of hands is particularly effective when praying for non-believers.

Anointing with Oil

Very closely associated with laying on of hands is the procedure of anointing the sick with oil and praying for healing. We find this admonition in James 5:14-15, which says:

> *"Is anyone among you sick? Let him call for the elders of the church, and let them pray over him, anointing him with oil in the name of the Lord; and the prayer offered in faith will restore the one who is sick, and the Lord will raise him up, and if he has committed sins, they will be forgiven him."*

These instructions were written to the church. Recognizing that many times the sick one is too weak to be able to stand on his own, the Lord has laid the responsibility for believing for healing and administering that healing, on the mature believers in any given body. The word *elder* here from the Greek actually means "older one" or "senior". Hopefully, the men who walk in the office of elder in churches are the senior or mature ones in the faith. But if you do not find that to be the case in your church body, do not hesitate to ask other believers whom you know to be mature in the Lord to anoint you with oil and pray for you. God will honor their prayers because they fulfill His requirements, regardless of chronological age or official title.

But remember, dear sick one, don't wait for the elders to come to you. It is your responsibility to call for them, for that is your act of faith.

The oil itself, of course, does not heal. But from the beginning of God's covenant relationships with man, anointing with oil has been a divinely ordained way of setting a person apart to the Lord. The priests of the old Covenant were consecrated in that way. The prophets of God anointed the kings of Israel in that way. So the oil applied to the sick one represents consecrating him to the Lord -- handing him completely over to the Lord, if you will, so that the Lord can work the deliverance and healing.

The sick one needs to realize that this act represents a true repentance for any sin not yet confessed, and a willingness to submit to God with his whole heart. Then, he comes into a place of receiving, as the elders release their faith to God, providing Him with an open channel through which to meet the sick one's need. Also, the oil, regardless of where it is applied, provides that very physical aid for the sufferer, which helps him release his faith at the very time of prayer and gives him a tangible experience on which to lean in any possible intervening spiritual battle over the manifestation.

As we said, it does not matter, of course, where the oil is applied unless the Lord leads specifically in a particular case. Over the years, it has been interesting to me as I have studied the ways in which others minister, as well as trying to be sensitive to what the Lord has directed me to do in ministering to the sick, that there are a variety of ways to anoint with oil. The priests of the Old Covenant often had the oil poured over their heads in such quantities that it ran down their shoulders and totally saturated their garments.

Generally, people praying for the sick take a small amount of oil and rub it rather inconspicuously on the forehead or, possibly, the affected part of the body. However, I often think of that great evangelist Smith Wigglesworth's testimony of how he went to pray for a woman near death. The minister who accompanied him and the woman's husband both prayed defeated, unbelieving prayers, at which point Wigglesworth began to feel desperate. His spirit responded to the magnitude of the woman's need with action of equal magnitude. He took a bottle full of oil from his back pocket and poured the entire contents out upon the woman's head, crying out to God to heal her, and He most certainly and immediately did so. No matter how it's done, beloved, the acts of faith and obedience in calling for the elders and anointing with oil will bring happy results.

The Lord's Supper / Holy Communion

When we partake of the Lord's Supper, or Holy Communion, we need to realize that we are coming into vital contact with Jesus Himself and should expect that something definite will happen to us for our good. The beauty of God's plan in instituting this meal of faith far surpasses what most churches allow for it. The meal itself is really only a part of the original Passover meal instituted the night before God led the Israelites out of Egypt. Therefore, in order to understand its power for us, we need to go back and look at the Passover carefully.

In Exodus, chapter 12, we have the story. The Lord instructed the Israelites to take an unblemished lamb, one per household, and slaughter it at twilight. They were warned not to break any bones in the lamb's body and to roast it that evening and eat it at once. Nor were they to leave any of it overnight; but must burn any leftovers. This action prohibited anyone not in relationship with God from partaking of the benefit of this sacrifice, which, of course, looked forward to Jesus. They were then to take hyssop and dip it into the blood of the lamb and apply it to the doorposts and lintels of their houses. All Israelites were to stay inside their houses, under the blood, if they would be spared. The Lord told them that the destroyer would come through the land of Egypt and kill every firstborn in Egypt – not just Egyptian firstborn – but **every** firstborn, both of man and livestock. The only escape from this plague was the one instituted by God Himself – the blood of the unspotted lamb on the door-posts. Anyone within the house covered by the applied blood was kept safe.

Notice that God did not give them a choice of avenues of escape that depended on their personal preferences; nor does He give us choices, beloved. If we want God's protection and help, we must follow His plan for receiving it or lose out.

All who followed the Lord's instructions were delivered from the plague of death that night, but that was not all of the Passover meal's benefit. Psalm 105:37 tells us that when He brought them out (the very next day) there was not one in the estimated two and a half to three million people who were sick or unable to travel. Let's read it right from God's Word: *"He brought them out with silver and gold; and among His tribes there was not one who stumbled."* That word **stumbled** in the Hebrew language means literally **"to be feeble, weak, cast down, or decayed"**. Praise God!

You know, beloved, that in the natural, a group of that size would have its share of people who were suffering from disease and degeneration of body, who would not be in any shape to make an exhausting trip like the one that lay before them. So there must have been something miraculous that took place from the time they partook of the lamb the previous evening to the time of departure. The blood broke the power of the plague and death, and the body of the lamb, blessed by God and eaten according to His exact instructions, imparted physical health and strength to these obedient people.

1 Corinthians 5:7 says, *"... For Christ **our Passover** also has been sacrificed."* Jesus Christ is considered the final Passover Lamb – the final sacrifice to break the power of the curse and death. The Lord told Israel that they were to celebrate the Passover meal as an everlasting celebration throughout all generations. When Jesus celebrated it with His disciples He explained that the elements of that meal, indeed the meal itself, was looking forward to His coming and completing the plan

of God for man's total deliverance; not just from Egypt, but from sin and all the curse that resulted from it.

If you take time to study the Passover meal, you find that certain elements, particularly a portion of bread and a glass of wine, were always set aside in recognition of the coming Messiah.   However, Jesus took these very elements and handed them to His disciples saying, as in Matthew 26:26-28: *"... Take, eat; this is My body,"* and *"Drink from it, all of you; for this is My blood of the covenant, which is poured out for many for forgiveness of sins."*

He's telling them that from now on, they won't partake of the Passover celebration to remember the great deliverance from Egypt, but to remember the finished work accomplished by Him for our ultimate deliverance from sin and all its evil consequences. Moreover, they are to believe that as they partake of the elements of the meal, they also partake, in a special way, of the powerful effects of His blood (which breaks the power of sin and its curse) and His body (which took our infirmities and carried away our diseases). That Body and Blood **have** overcome, and bring to each of us that same victory.

That is why the Lord moved on St. Paul to write in 1 Corinthians 11:27-30:

> *"Therefore whoever eats the bread or drinks the cup of the Lord in an unworthy manner, shall be guilty of the body and the blood of the Lord. But let a man examine himself, and so let him eat of the bread and drink of the cup. For he who eats and drinks, eats and drinks judgment to himself,*

if he does not judge the body rightly. **For this reason many among you are weak and sick, and a number sleep (die)."**

Many Christians mistakenly think that when the Word refers here to judging or discerning the body rightly, that it means discerning the body of believers – the church – as the body of Christ. However, that is not the case. In the following chapter of 1 Corinthians, reference is made to the body of believers being recognized. But in these verses, the Lord is referring to the actual physical body of Christ that was sacrificed for us.

Note verse 27 again. If we fail to acknowledge that in this meal we are coming into vital contact with that body and blood and its accomplished work, we are **guilty of both the body and blood of the Lord Himself**. And then verse 30 extends the instruction by saying that many are sick and dying early because they have failed this acknowledgment.

It is an understatement to say that this is not an experience to trifle with. It carries within it the power of life and death. The Word speaks of examining or judging ourselves before we partake. That does not mean, dear believer, that we are to see all of our shortcomings and sins and say we are just too unworthy to partake. No, not at all. We are to see our sins, but we **are** to see the glorious power in the body and blood offered for us to wipe out those sins and their power over us.

We can't make ourselves worthy to receive the Lord's Supper. But acknowledging that we need it so desperately and that it embodies the elements that worked our deliverance from sin, the world, and our flesh, is what makes us **ready** to partake of it and all its merits. When we come to the Lord's table, we must be sure that we believe that **He** is there and that these elements bring the real power of His death and resurrection to us – spirit, soul, and body. Some of the people of Corinth were sick and dying because they were eating this meal just like they would any other. They were ignoring the presence of the very God Himself, Who worked their salvation.

The other side of this coin is that when we truly believe and receive in this meal the Lord Jesus Himself and the full effect of His sacrificed, resurrected body and blood, we can receive into ourselves all that was purchased for us by Him – not the least of which is healing. There have been times in my experience, when I believed God for physical healing and felt led to partake of the Lord's Supper in sweet communion with the Lord alone. I took my unleavened bread and wine and went apart by myself with the Lord. I meditated on what the Word says His body and blood have accomplished for me, and I prayed that He would meet me at that very moment with a special releasing of those blessings. I have never failed to experience results in those cases. I have done the same at times when I needed healing in my soul also, with equal benefit.

I know believers who have been led to partake of the Lord's Supper every day, or several times a day, for a period of time, while seeking healing from the Lord, only to have the full benefits of His body and blood manifested in their flesh as a result. Many have been the testimonies, also, of believers who had been holding onto the Lord for some time for the miracle they needed, and during communion service at church, as they truly perceived the presence of the Lord, they received their healing need met.

This is not some formula, beloved. But this is one of the many avenues God has provided for us to be able to release our faith and receive from Him. As we have said before, everything of God has healing and life in it. You must draw close to the Lord and let His Spirit lead you into which avenue or combination of avenues will bring the manifestation of your miracle.

Praying for Others

James 5:16 says, *"... confess your sins to one another, and pray for one another, so that you may be healed."* I believe that praying for one another releases healing, not only to the one for whom prayer is being made, but also to the one doing the praying. It is part of God's beautiful plan that each of our unselfish and loving acts puts a spiritual law into operation that brings something good back to us. So it is with prayer made on behalf of another. When we pray in love and faith for someone else, not only does this spiritual law go into operation for us, but we also move into a position of complete openness to God. When interceding for another, we open all the channels and make personal contact with the power of God that delivers and heals. Many people find at these times that their own need for healing, which **seemed** to stubbornly resist former prayers, is suddenly met by God's power.

Although I have known of numerous instances when this kind of blessing occurred, the one that is most memorable to me concerns a friend who, several years ago, suffered from a debilitating, life-shortening disease called Myasthenia Gravis. She had suffered for a long time and was growing worse. She and her husband, after learning of God's will for healing, prayed and sought ministry for her healing. They continued to hold on to the Lord in spite of the symptoms growing worse.

Then one evening, they received a request to pray for another lady who was seriously ill. While reaching out to the Lord in faith for this lady, my friend experienced the miraculous move of God upon her own body. She began to improve dramatically from that day forward and progressed to perfect health, which she was still experiencing a year later when I came to know her. Praise God! When you are sick, that's an excellent time to exercise your faith for others.

Praying in Tongues

Many people do not realize that the ability to pray in tongues is also a very valuable tool when seeking healing from the Lord. Of course, this gift comes with the baptism in the Holy Spirit. Unfortunately, because so many in the Body of Christ have been taught that the baptism in the Holy Spirit and tongues are not for today, those Christians do not have the opportunity to take advantage of this avenue to health.

It is not the purpose of this book to teach a lesson on tongues, so we will limit the explanation to the following: There are two different categories of tongues spoken of in the Word of God. One is the gift described in 1 Corinthians 12, which includes both tongues for personal prayer and for giving messages from the Lord in public meetings.

When used for giving public messages, the tongues must be accompanied by interpretation, and scripture explains that tongues used in that category are not necessarily available to everyone all the time. The gift of tongues for messages, along with the gift of interpretation are operated, like all the other nine gifts of the Spirit, and they are manifested only as the Spirit wills. The entire chapter of 1 Corinthians 14 gives detailed explanations of how these gifts should be used in public meetings.

However, the second category – tongues for personal use – is given to all believers and, whether or not those believers make use this gift is entirely up to each person. We must be careful to understand that even if we do not find ourselves used to give public messages in tongues, we have Jesus' word of promise that we will have access to tongues for personal prayer equally with every other believer. Mark 16:15-17 tells us clearly,

> *"Go into all the world and preach the gospel to all creation. He who has believed and has been baptized shall be saved. ... And these signs will accompany those who have believed: In My name, they will cast out demons; they will speak with new tongues."*

Now, the word translated in English as "tongues" is actually the Greek word which means "languages not learned through natural means." So, in other words, a totally supernatural gift from the Lord that bypasses our intellect.

The Lord explains, through the words of St. Paul, in Romans 8:2-27, that often *"we do not know how to pray as we should."* And, of course, many people, when they are suffering physically, find it hard to pray as effectively as they need to pray. But God has a solution to this problem, and verse 26 tells us that His Holy Spirit helps us pray through utterances too deep for words. (The literal Greek here says "groanings or utterances too deep for articulate speech.")

St. Paul, through the Holy Spirit, goes on to tell us in 1 Corinthians 14:5 that he wishes we would all pray much in tongues. And he makes clear in verse 14 of that chapter that when we pray in tongues, our minds are not involved – only our spirits. It is true that our minds must make the decision to allow our spirit to be in charge of our prayer, so that we release our tongue to speak the utterances the Holy Spirit gives us, but other than making that decision of the will, the mind has no part to play. As a result of that fact, our own mind, our own lack of understanding of medical conditions, and our own fears are shut out, and our spirit – helped by the Holy Spirit – takes over our prayers.

But possibly one of the most exciting truths in this passage of Scripture is what we learn in verses 2 and 4 of chapter 14. Verse 2 tells us that when we pray in tongues, we speak mysteries to God. He can also speak mysteries back to us because He's in charge of the language. We

119

must do the actual physical speaking, but He provides what's being said in the sounds we make. But since we're speaking mysteries, not only does our un-renewed mind stay out of the picture, but so does the enemy of our souls, because he can't understand what we're saying either.

But wait: It still gets better. Verse 4 tells us that the one who prays in tongues edifies himself. Now, most people consider that verse to mean that we build ourselves up spiritually. And, of course, we do, but that's not the total benefit. The word translated "edify" means "to build or repair the house." Now, let that sink in: your spirit is praying (with the language provided by the Holy Spirit), and that prayer is building or repairing your spirit's house. And what is that house? That's right – it's your physical body. A number of Christians have learned that healing – especially for seriously troubling or obstinate maladies – can come successfully through praying in tongues.

The Word As Medicine

The final means of healing that we will look at is the one that probably excites me the most. Our dear Great Physician does not need a pharmacy. He has created one medicine for us, and It will accomplish a complete cure for any illness or infirmity of body or mind. It has absolutely no negative side effects. It has no expiration date, and It will never drain our finances. God's medicine is His very own Word.

Psalm 107:20 says,
"He sent His Word and healed them."

Proverbs 4:20-22 says:
"My son, give attention to my words; incline thine heart unto my sayings. Let them not depart from thine eyes; keep them in the midst of thine heart. For they are life to those who find them and health to their whole body."

The word **health** here is the Hebrew word for **medicine**. So we have a promise here that the very words spoken by God will work on our flesh like physical medicine. I once heard a minister giving testimony of how he became convinced that God had made provision for healing His people. He said that this one Scripture did the most to help him, because it was one healing Scripture that no one could spiritualize by insisting that it did not refer to physical healing.

The Word of God is able to change our flesh, of course, because it was that very Word that created the matter out of which our flesh is made. Hebrews 4:12 says:

"The Word of God is living and active, sharper than any two-edged sword, and piercing as far as the division of soul and spirit, of both joints and morrow ..."

How interesting that it enters into the very morrow of our body. That is the root source of our blood and cell production. Can you see that the Word in the very manufacturing center of a human body can completely remake that whole body?

How do we get It to work? The more we study the Word, meditate on It, and speak It out of our mouth, the more It works Its way into our whole system, producing Its life there. However, when we are facing a specific physical problem, we can take doses of this priceless medicine just like we do a prescription from a human doctor. I have done this so often and know of numerous testimonies of other believers who have done the same. Taking the Word of God as medicine has cured migraine headaches, kidney infections, paralysis from strokes, broken bones, cancer, tuberculosis, mental deficiencies, and multitudes of other illnesses of body and soul.

Find the healing Scriptures that relate to your particular malady, or the ones that speak particularly to your heart, and begin to read them or speak them to your body. Put your own name into them. You may need to take a dose three or four times a day. In a particularly critical case, I have known believers to read their Scriptures every fifteen minutes for several days. I know of one testimony in which a lady with tuberculosis read, or listened to the reading, of Scriptures referring to her condition almost constantly for several days. She was almost dead and virtually without faith for healing when another believer began reading the Scriptures to her. She gradually became strong enough to read for herself, and the Word Itself created faith in her heart. Suddenly, one day, the reality of her healing exploded in her heart, and she jumped from her bed completely healed.

Probably the most precious testimony from my own life in this regard concerns a time when my husband was experiencing some very alarming physical problems. One day he suddenly began having severe chest pain and feeling extremely weak and sleepy. By the next day, he could hardly stay awake at all, and when he was awake, his speech was sluggish and slurred. I prayed and called on several other believers for agreeing prayer. The symptoms persisted, and Richard lay in bed, almost constantly asleep. He was unable to stay up and alert for any lengthy periods.

As I sat beside his bed on the worst day, praying and speaking the Word, the Lord quickened to me His Word from Psalm 118: 16-17. I grasped it like a life preserver, which it was. I put Richard's name into the Scripture and began to speak it to him: *"The right hand of the Lord does valiantly. Richard shall not die, but live, and tell of the works of the Lord."* I realized that this one verse had everything in it that he needed at the time. It covered his need for life to drive out death, which was obviously at work, and his need for complete restoration of his speaking faculties.

I spoke that Word to him consistently throughout the day, whether he was waking or sleeping. I sat beside the bed for long periods of time, speaking it over and over and over. By the next day, he showed definite improvement. I continued to speak God's Word, and he continued to improve. By the following week, he was back to normal and has never had a recurrence of the problem in the six years since that time.

One of the most rapid healings I ever received personally by applying the Word as medicine was for an abscessed tooth. I awoke early one morning with severe pain in and around a broken tooth in my upper right jaw. I couldn't stand to eat on it, so I had something warm to drink, took a dose of the most potent pain killer I could buy over the counter, and went on to work. I also took along a bottle of medication to apply topically to my tooth and gums. You may ask, "Didn't you pray?" Yes, I did pray, but it was more or less on the run. I was blessed to be teaching in a Christian school, so I asked for prayer at work also.

However, by the time my first class was over, the pain was going all over my jaw, up the whole right side of my head, and part way down my neck. It was the most excruciating, indescribable pain I'd ever experienced. I applied and reapplied the topical medication, with no appreciable benefit at all. I took a second dose of pain medicine as soon as the time limit on the bottle would allow – again with no effect. By 11:30 that morning, the pain had become so debilitating that I could no longer function at work, so I went home – barely able to concentrate on my driving. I had a strong conviction in my heart that if I could just close myself away with the Word of God for a while, I would receive my healing.

My husband and a friend were working on the television antenna when I arrived home. Aware of the oddity of my coming home at that time of day, my husband followed me into the house to see what was wrong. As I told him, I was already getting into bed and putting a tape of healing Scriptures into the tape recorder on my nightstand. He prayed for me briefly and went back outside to finish his work. I turned on the tape of healing Scriptures and began to let my spirit and body absorb their medicine. I fell asleep listening to the Word. I awoke about an hour later with all of the pain completely gone. I was able to eat on that tooth and do whatever I liked, totally free from pain. The Word of God had done what God had sent it to do.

A few years ago, my husband had a broken hip that would not seem to heal. For a period of three or four months, the doctors could see no indication of improvement in the bones at all. The orthopedic surgeon said tests indicated the bones were failing to get proper blood supply, due to other tissue damage caused by the break. But we faithfully spoke the Word of God to those bones and blood vessels. We took Scriptures of healing, especially some relating specifically to bones, and applied them in faith for months. We also prayed, of course, and many strong believers in our church and family also prayed for us faithfully. The enemy tried to discourage us. He tried to convince us that after so much time had passed, even God's Word would not cause healing to begin again.

But, dear Christian, the devil is a liar, and God is faithful to His Word. That holy medicine worked itself into my husband's bones and produced healing. All of a sudden, those bones began to knit together properly by the power of God, and in every examination that followed, the doctor was able to report that he saw no indication of problems with the blood supply to those bones. It was sweet victory when the doctor was able to look at the x-rays and tell Richard that his hip was completely healed. (Knowing that this was one of those times when Richard and I felt the need for some human medical help also, the Lord graciously led us to a doctor who continually encouraged us to keep praying and believing God for our miracle. He knew also that the outcome lay in God's hands alone.)

Another very encouraging testimony of healing through application of the Word concerns a friend of mine who is a praise and worship leader and a very active leader in the Women's Aglow organization. She had been having serious problems with high blood pressure. She went to the doctor, who put her on medication, but it just wouldn't bring the pressure down. Finally the doctor decided to send her to the local hospital for a special shot that would make her pressure go down rapidly. For a few minutes after she had taken the shot, everything seemed to be all right, and the nurse left her alone to rest a few minutes before going home. Suddenly she began having an allergic reaction to the drug in the shot. Her left arm became numb. Then her heart began to pound as if it would come out of her body.

By the time her daughter had brought the nurse and doctor to the room, my friend's whole body was completely out of control. She said that her mind still worked, but all it would do was tell her she was going to die. She was able to speak periodically to the doctor at first, but finally even speaking became more than she could handle. She could hear the nurse talking to her daughter about a rash that had broken out on her body, and she could tell that they were hooking her up to some monitoring devices. The other thing she could understand was that the doctor himself was very alarmed, and, naturally, fear began to work on her too.

Her daughter had called other believers to pray, and, before long, my friend's pastor came in. She was still in this crisis situation and said that, by this time, she could feel herself sinking farther and farther down. Her pastor walked to her bedside, laid his hand on her head, and began **singing** the Word from Isaiah 60:1: *"Arise, shine, for thy light is come, and the glory of the Lord is risen upon thee."*

She said he sang this song over and over and over, and as he did, she could feel her spirit respond. She began to feel herself being drawn back up, up, up. She was so aware that the power in that Scripture song was what was drawing her back to normalcy that she said although she couldn't talk at this time, she kept thinking, "Don't stop. Don't stop singing." Her faithful pastor, led by God, kept singing, and everything in her body gradually came back to normal. The pastor himself later related that he had never been led to minister in just that way before, but all he felt to do was to sing her that Word. That precious Word! It heals and brings life when nothing else can!

I'll close this chapter with one final personal testimony. A few years ago, I began having a lot of pain in my throat and upper chest. I assumed it was some kind of viral thing that was trying to get a place in my body and began to resist it, based on my authority from the Word of God. I enforced the law of the spirit of life against it. However, the symptoms didn't leave immediately, and being really busy with work, I just sort of let the thing drag on without really standing my ground.

127

By a couple days later, I realized the pain was still there and actually a little worse, so I finally paid enough attention to actually pray about it. When it still persisted, I had my husband pray, and then a couple other family members. But by two weeks into the situation, with the symptoms getting worse – even debilitating by this time – I realized I had to get alone with the Lord and find out what the problem was.

So I went to church one morning where I could be alone with God and totally focused on Him. I got down before Him and said, "Lord I *know* you have given me the deliverance and healing that I'm in need of. And *You* know that I know You've granted it to me. But I'm not receiving the manifestation. I need more help. Please help me. Show me what to do."

I sat there quietly for a while, and the Lord sat quietly as well. I thought about the fact that God had taught me long ago that I needed to use His Word as medicine, but I had been negligent in that respect this time. So I prayed again:

"Father, I know I need to take Your Word as medicine, but could you give me a specific prescription for this particular thing that will make me able to receive the whole manifestation?" I felt assurance in my heart that He was more than willing to do that, so I said, "I'll just pray in the Spirit and believe you to show me exactly which scriptures to read for this problem."

I proceeded to pray in tongues for a while, resting in the belief that the Lord would be revealing to my mind the scriptures to read. In a short time, I began to hear in my mind the chapters and verses of specific passages from the Word. I stopped praying in tongues and made note of the scripture references.

Then I said, "Okay, Father, I'll read these verses, but how often should I take this prescription?"

The answer rose up in my spirit immediately: "Once an hour for seven hours."

I received that prescription and took the first dose right then. My husband and I had some errands to do in a neighboring town, so he drove, and I took my Bible along so that I could read my prescription every hour while we were gone. Now this condition had been with me for over two weeks, getting worse the whole time. But by the time I had read those scripture the fourth time, the symptoms had lessened to half. And by the time I had read all seven hours they were so minimal that I was only barely aware of them. I went to bed in total peace, and awoke completely well.

Dear sick one, if we will be as faithful to apply God's medicine to our physical bodies as we are the prescriptions from a human doctor, we will get the most wonderful results. Even people who aren't sure they believe have found that by applying the Word with an honest heart, the faith has been created in them by the Word itself, and then the physical results come. So open up God's Medicine Chest. Read the Word. Sing it. Play it on tape. Have others read it to you. Use any or all methods of getting this divine medicine into your being. For whatever the diagnosis, the Word of God is the cure.

Questions for Review:

1. God has only one remedy of His own for all sickness. What is that remedy?

2. Is God displeased with us if we feel we need to make use of the treatments medical science offers?

3. In order to have faith to pray for our own healing effectively, what must we abide in?

4. What Scripture is a particular encouragement for husbands and wives to pray together?

5. Whom does God consider the high priest of the home?

6. Name one example in Scripture where an individual received his healing gradually as hands were laid on him more than once.

7. According to James 5:14-15, when a person is too sick to stand on his own faith for his healing, upon whom does God place the responsibility for believing for and administering that healing?

8. Anointing with oil has long been a divinely appointed way of doing what?

9. What we know as the Lord's Supper is actually part of what original meal?

10. Corinthians 11:27 says that anyone who eats the bread and drinks the cup of the Lord's Supper in an unworthy manner shall be guilty of what?

11. What Scripture tells us that God's Word is medicine for our flesh?

Questions for Meditation and Discussion:

1. What is the difference between the unbelievers in Jesus' hometown for whom He could work no major miracles and a believer with weak faith? How do we increase our faith?

2. Do you think anointing with oil is an important practice that should continue to be carried out in the modern church? Why?

3. Corinthians 11 says that some people were getting sick and dying early because they were not receiving the Lord's Supper properly. That means that partaking of this meal is a life and death matter. How is that so and why? How can we be sure to avoid that problem in our own life so that we receive only life and healing from that meal?

4. How can praying for others help us receive our own healing?

5. How does God's Word work as medicine in our bodies and bring healing?

GOD'S MEDICINE CHEST

In the previous chapter, we talked about God's Word being one of the means He uses to heal us. It is His medicine, and as we take it into our system, we can be assured that it will do what He promised: produce health and life in our whole being. There are hundreds of Scriptures that contain God's life and health in them, but the following are some of the most powerful that I have used in my own experience and have known to be effective in other believers' lives as well.

I have listed many of them categorically, under the headings of some of the most common diseases and problems. However, please do not feel that you need to use only those listed in each category. Most of these Scriptures apply to numerous problems, and, of course, some (especially those listed in the "General" category) can be applied to all healing needs.

Choose the ones that relate to your situation, or use them all. Read them daily, or many times a day, depending on how you feel led in your own spirit. You might also ask the Lord to show you other verses from His Word that will help you particularly. Don't forget to put your own name in them, or the name of your loved one, and read them aloud.

Addictions & Sicknesses Known to
Have a Demonic Spirit at the Root

♦ **Matthew 8:16-17:** And when evening had come, they brought to Him many who were demon-possessed; and He cast out the spirits with a word, and healed all who were ill in order that what was spoken through Isaiah the prophet might be fulfilled, saying, "He Himself took our infirmities, and carried away our diseases."

♦ **Matthew 8:18:** Verily I say unto you; Whatsoever ye shall bind on earth shall be bound in heaven; and whatsoever ye shall loose on earth shall be loosed in heaven. (KJV).

♦ **Isaiah 49:24-25:** Can the prey be taken from the mighty man, or the captives of a tyrant be rescued?" Surely, thus says the Lord, "Even the captives of the mighty man will be taken away, and the prey of the tyrant will be rescued; for I will contend with the one who contends with you..."

♦ **2 Cor. 10:4-5:** For though we walk in the flesh, we do not war according to the flesh, for the weapons of our warfare are not of the flesh, but divinely powerful for the destruction of fortresses.

♦ **Revelation 12:11:** And they overcame him (the devil) by the blood of the Lamb, and by the word of their testimony. (KJV).

♦ **Habakkuk 3:13:** Thou didst go forth for the salvation of Thy people. For the salvation of Thine anointed. Thou didst strike the head of the house of the evil to lay him open from thigh to neck.

♦ **1 John 3:8b:** For this purpose was the Son of God manifested, that He might destroy the works of the devil.

♦ **John 8:36:** If the Son therefore shall make you free, you shall be free indeed.

♦ **Psalm 107:17-20:** Fools because of their rebellious way, and because of their iniquities, were afflicted. Their soul abhorred all kinds of food; and they drew near to the gates of death. They cried out to the Lord in their trouble; He saved them out of their distresses. He sent His word and healed them, and delivered them from their destruction.

♦ **Rom. 8:2:** For the law of the Spirit of life in Christ Jesus has set you free from the law of sin and of death.

AIDS (Acquired Immune Deficiency Syndrome)

♦ **Psalm 103:1-5:** Bless the Lord, O my soul, and all that is within me, bless His holy name. Bless the Lord, O my soul, and forget none of His benefits; Who forgiveth all thine iniquities, Who healeth all thy diseases; Who redeemeth thy life from destruction; Who crowneth thee with lovingkindness and tender mercies; Who satisfieth thy mouth with good things; so that thy youth is renewed like the eagle's. (KJV).

♦ **Psalm 107:17-20:** Fools because of their rebellious way, and because of their iniquities, were afflicted. Their soul abhorred all kinds of food; and they drew near to the gates of death. They cried out to the Lord in their trouble; He saved them out of their distresses. He sent His word and healed them, and delivered them from their destruction.

♦ **Psalm 27:1-2:** The Lord is my light and my salvation; whom shall I fear? The Lord is the defense of my life; whom shall I dread: When evildoers came upon me to devour my flesh, my adversaries and my enemies, they stumbled and fell.

♦ **Matthew 8:16-17:** And when evening had come, they brought to Him many who were demon-possessed; and He cast out the spirits with a word, and healed all who were ill in order that what was spoken through

Isaiah the prophet might be fulfilled, saying, "He Himself took our infirmities, and carried away our diseases."

♦ **1 John 3:8b:** For this purpose was the Son of God manifested, that He might destroy the works of the devil.

♦ **John 8:36:** If the Son therefore shall make you free, you shall be free indeed.

Alzheimer's and Other Mental Diseases and Infirmities

♦ **2 Timothy 1:7:** For God hath not given us the spirit of fear; but of power, and of love, and of a sound mind. (KJV).

♦ **1 Cor. 1:16b:** But we have the mind of Christ.

♦ **Isaiah 50:7a:** For the Lord will help me; therefore shall I not be confounded.

♦ **2 Cor. 10:4-5:** For the weapons of our warfare are not carnal, but mighty through God to the pulling down of strongholds; casting down imaginations, and every high thing that exalteth itself against the knowledge of God, and bringing into captivity every thought to the obedience of Christ. (KJV).

♦ **Philippians 4:6-7:** Be anxious for nothing, but in everything by prayer and supplication with thanksgiving let your requests be made known to God. And the peace of God, which surpasses all comprehension, shall guard your hearts and your minds in Christ Jesus.

♦ **Philippians 4:8:** Finally, brethren, whatever is true, whatever is honorable, whatever is right, whatever is pure, whatever is lovely, whatever is of good repute, if there is any excellence and if anything worthy of praise, let your mind dwell on these things.

♦ **Proverbs 16:3:** Commit thy works unto the Lord, and thy thoughts shall be established.

♦ **Isaiah 26:3:** Thou wilt keep him in perfect peace, whose mind is stayed on Thee: because he trusteth in Thee. (KJV).

♦ **Romans 8:6:** For the mind set on the flesh in death, but the mind set on the Spirit is life and peace.

♦ **Hebrews 10:16:** This is the covenant that I will make with them after those days, says the Lord: I will put My laws upon their heart, and upon their mind I will write them.

Arthritis & Other Crippling Diseases

♦ **Malachi 4:2:** But for you who fear My name the sun of righteousness will rise with healing in its wings; and you will go forth and skip about like calves from the stall.

♦ **Mark 11:22b-25:** Have faith in God. Truly I say to you, whoever says to this mountain, "Be taken up and cast into the sea," and does not doubt in his heart, but believes that what he says is going to happen, it shall be granted him. Therefore I say to you, all things for which you pray and ask, believe that you have received them, and they shall be granted to you. And whenever you stand praying, forgive, if you have anything against anyone; so that your Father also who is in heaven may forgive you your transgressions.

♦ **1 Cor. 6:19-20:** Or do you not know that your body is a temple of the Holy Spirit who is in you, whom you have from God, and that you are not your own? For you have been bought with a price: therefore glorify God in your body.

♦ **Matt. 15:30-31:** And great multitudes came to Him, bringing with them those who were lame, crippled, blind, dumb, and many others, and they laid them down at His feet; and He healed them, so that the multitude marveled as they saw the dumb speaking, the crippled restored, and the lame walking, and the blind seeing; and they glorified the God of Israel.

♦ **Psalm 145:14:** The Lord upholdeth all that fall and raiseth up all those that be bowed down.

♦ **Matthew 8:17:** "He Himself took our infirmities, and carried away our diseases."

♦ **Romans 8:11:** But if the Spirit of Him who raised Jesus from the dead dwells in you, He who raised Christ Jesus from the dead will give life to your mortal bodies through His Spirit who indwells you.

Blood Diseases

♦ **Leviticus 17:11:** For the life of the flesh is in the blood, and I have given it to you on the altar to make atonement for your souls.

♦ **Joel 3:21:** For I will cleanse their blood that I have not cleansed: for the Lord dwelleth in Zion.

♦ **Ezekiel 16:6:** " ... I said to you while you were in your blood, 'Live!'. I said to you while you were in your blood, 'Live!'."

♦ **Matt. 26:27-28:** And He took the cup and gave thanks, and gave it to them, saying, "Drink from it all of you; for this is My blood of the covenant, which is to be shed on behalf of many for forgiveness of sins."

♦ **Revelation 12:11:** And they overcame him (the devil) by the blood of the Lamb, and by the word of their testimony. (KJV).

♦ **Romans 8:2:** For the law of the Spirit of life in Christ Jesus has set you free from the law of sin and of death.

Bone Problems

♦ **Psalm 34:19-20:** Many are the afflictions of the righteous; but the Lord delivers him out of them all. He keeps all his bones; not one of them is broken.

♦ **Proverbs 3:7-8:** Do not by wise in your own eyes; reverently fear and worship the Lord, and turn away from evil. It shall be health to your nerves and sinews, and morrow and moistening to your bones. (Amplified).

♦ **Proverbs 16:24:** Pleasant words are as an honeycomb, sweet to the soul, and health to the bones.

♦ **Isaiah 58:9b-11:** If you remove the yoke from your midst, the pointing of the finger, and speaking wickedness, and if you give yourself to the hungry, and satisfy the desire of the afflicted, then your light will rise in darkness, and your gloom will become like midday. And the Lord will continually guide you, and satisfy your desire in scorched places, and give strength to your bones.

♦ **Ezekiel 37:5-6:** Thus saith the Lord God unto these bones; "Behold, I will cause breath to enter into you, and ye shall live: and I will lay sinews upon you, and will bring up flesh upon you, and cover you with skin, and put breath in you, and ye shall live; and ye shall know that I am the Lord. (KJV).

♦ **Malachi 4:2:** But for you who fear My name the sun of righteousness will rise with healing in its wings; and you will go forth and skip about like calves from the stall.

♦ **Psalm 35:9-10:** And my soul shall rejoice in the Lord; it shall exult in His salvation. All my bones will say, "Lord, who is like Thee, who delivers the afflicted from him who is too strong for him, and the afflicted and the needy from him who robs him?"

♦ **Hebrews 4:12:** For the word of God is quick and powerful and sharper than a two-edged sword, piercing even to the dividing asunder of soul and spirit, and of the joints and morrow.

♦ **Ephesians 5:30:** For we are members of his body, of his flesh, and of his bones.

Broken Hearts

♦ **Psalm 147:3:** He heals the brokenhearted, and binds up their wounds.

♦ **Isaiah 61:1-3:** The Spirit of the Lord God is upon me, because the Lord has anointed me to bring good news to the afflicted; He has sent me to bind up the brokenhearted, to proclaim the favorable year of the Lord, ... to comfort all who mourn, to grant those who mourn in Zion, giving them a garland instead of ashes, the oil of gladness instead of mourning, the mantle of praise instead of a spirit of fainting.

♦ **Psalm 30:5b:** Weeping may last for the night, but a shout of joy comes in the morning.

♦ **Psalm 30:11:** Thou hast turned for me my mourning into dancing; thou hast loosed my sackcloth and girded me with gladness; that my soul may sing praise to you and not be silent. O Lord my God, I will give thanks to Thee forever.

♦ **Isaiah 53:4-5:** Surely He has borne our griefs – sickness, weakness and distress -- and carried our sorrows and pain. ... He was wounded for our transgressions, He was bruised for our guilt and iniquities; the chastisement needful to obtain peace and well-being for us was upon Him, and with the stripes that wounded Him we are healed and made whole. (Amplified).

♦ **Psalm 42:5:** Why are you in despair, O my soul? And why have you become disturbed within me? Hope in God, for I shall again praise Him for the help of His presence.

♦ **Acts 2:28:** Thou hast made known to me the ways of life; Thou wilt make me full of gladness with Thy presence.

Cancer -- Growths – Tumors

♦ **Psalm 27:1-2:** The Lord is my light and my salvation; whom shall I fear? The Lord is the defense of my life; whom shall I dread: When evildoers came upon me to devour my flesh, my adversaries and my enemies, they stumbled and fell.

♦ **Psalm 118:16-17:** The right hand of the Lord is exalted; The right hand of the Lord does valiantly. I shall not die, but live, and tell of the works of the Lord.

♦ **Matthew 15:13:** But He answered and said, "Every plant which My heavenly Father did not plant shall be rooted up."

♦ **Mark 11:22b-25:** Have faith in God. Truly I say to you, whoever says to this mountain, "Be taken up and cast into the sea," and does not doubt in his heart, but believes that what he says is going to happen, it shall be granted him. Therefore I say to you, all things for which you pray and ask, believe that you have received them, and they shall be granted to you. And whenever you stand praying, forgive, if you have anything against anyone; so that your Father also who is in heaven may forgive you your transgressions.

♦ **Matthew 18:18:** Verily I say unto you; Whatsoever ye shall bind on earth shall be bound in heaven; and whatsoever ye shall loose on earth shall be loosed in heaven. (KJV).

♦ **Matthew 8:16-17:** And when evening had come, they brought to Him many who were demon-possessed; and He cast out the spirits with a word, and healed all who were ill in order that what was spoken through Isaiah the prophet might be fulfilled, saying, "He Himself took our infirmities, and carried away our diseases."

♦ **Psalm 103:1-5:** Bless the Lord, O my soul, and all that is within me, bless His holy name. Bless the Lord, O my soul, and forget none of His benefits; Who forgiveth all thine iniquities, Who healeth all thy diseases; Who redeemeth thy life from destruction; Who crowneth thee with lovingkindness and tender mercies; Who satisfieth thy mouth with good things; so that thy youth is renewed like the eagle's. (KJV).

♦ **Psalm 107:17-20:** Fools because of their rebellious way, and because of their iniquities, were afflicted. Their soul abhorred all kinds of food; and they drew near to the gates of death. They cried out to the Lord in their trouble; He saved them out of their distresses. He sent His word and healed them, and delivered them from their destruction.

♦ **Romans 8:2:** For the law of the Spirit of life in Christ Jesus has set you free from the law of sin and of death.

Diseases & Disorders Associated with Aging

♦ **Isaiah 46:4:** Even to your old age, I shall be the same, and even to your graying years I shall bear you! I have done it, and I shall carry you; and I shall bear you, and I shall deliver you.

♦ **Psalm 103:1-5:** Bless the Lord, O my soul, and all that is within me, bless His holy name. Bless the Lord, O my soul, and forget none of His benefits; Who forgiveth all thine iniquities, Who healeth all thy diseases; Who redeemeth thy life from destruction; Who crowneth thee with lovingkindness and tender mercies; Who satisfieth thy mouth with good things; so that thy youth is renewed like the eagle's. (KJV).

♦ **Psalm 71:18:** And even when I am old and gray, O God, do not forsake me, until I declare Thy strength to this generation, Thy power to all who are to come.

♦ **Psalm 92:12-14:** The righteous man will flourish like the palm tree; he will grow like a cedar in Lebanon. Planted in the house of the Lord, they will flourish in the courts of our God. They will still yield fruit in old age; they shall be full of sap and very green, to declare that the Lord is upright; He is my rock, and there is no unrighteousness in Him.

Eye – Ear – Tongue Problems

♦ **Proverbs 20:12:** The hearing ear and the seeing eye, the Lord has made both of them.

♦ **Psalm 19:8b:** The commandment of the Lord is pure, enlightening the eyes.

♦ **Psalm 146:8a:** The Lord openeth the eyes of the blind ....

♦ **Luke 18:42:** And Jesus said to him, "Receive your sight; your faith has made you well."

♦ **Matthew 11:4-5:** And Jesus answered and said to them, "Go and report to John the things which you hear and see: the blind receive sight and the lame walk, the lepers are cleansed and the deaf hear, and the dead are raised up, and the poor have the gospel preached to them.

♦ **Job 36:15:** He delivereth the poor in his affliction, and openeth their ears in oppression.

♦ **Mark 7:34b-35:** He (Jesus) said to him, "Ephphatha!" that is, "Be opened!" and his ears were opened and the impediment of his tongue was removed, and he began speaking plainly.

♦ **Mark 7:37b:** He has done all things well; He makes even the deaf to hear, and the dumb to speak.

♦ **Matt. 15:30-31:** And great multitudes came to Him, bringing with them those who were lame, crippled, blind, dumb, and many others, and they laid them down at His feet; and He healed them, so that the multitude marveled as they saw the dumb speaking, the crippled restored, and the lame walking, and the blind seeing; and they glorified the God of Israel.

Headaches and Head Injuries

♦ **Psalm 3:3:** But Thou, O Lord, art a shield about me; my glory and the One who lifts my head.

♦ **Psalm 140:7:** O God, the Lord, the strength of my salvation, Thou hast covered my head in the day of battle.

♦ **Isaiah 53:4-5:** Surely He has borne our griefs – sickness, weakness and distress – and carried our sorrows and pain. ... He was wounded for our transgressions, He was bruised for our guilt and iniquities; the chastisement needful to obtain peace and well being for us was upon Him, and with the stripes that wounded Him we are healed and made whole. (Amplified).

♦ **Proverbs 14:30:** A tranquil heart is life to the body.

♦ **John 14:27a:** Peace I leave with you, My peace I give unto you.

Heart & Circulatory Problems

♦ **Psalm 73:26:** My flesh and my heart may fail; but God is the strength of my heart and my portion forever.

♦ **Psalm 27:14:** Wait upon the Lord; be of good courage, and He shall strengthen thine heart. (KJV).

♦ **Psalm 28:7:** The Lord is my strength and my shield; my heart trusts in Him, and I am helped.

♦ **Proverbs 17:22:** A joyful heart is good medicine.

♦ **Romans 8:2:** For the law of the Spirit of life in Christ Jesus has set you free from the law of sin and of death.

♦ **Romans 8:11:** But if the Spirit of Him who raised Jesus from the dead dwells in you, He who raised Christ Jesus from the dead will give life to your mortal bodies through His Spirit who indwells you.

♦ **Malachi 4:2:** But for you who fear My name the sun of righteousness will rise with healing in its wings; and you will go forth and skip about like calves from the stall.

♦ **Matthew 8:17b:** He Himself took our infirmities, and carried away our diseases.

♦ **Philippians 4:6-7:** Be anxious for nothing, but in everything by prayer and supplication with thanksgiving let your requests be made known to God. And the peace of God, which surpasses all comprehension, shall guard your hearts and your minds in Christ Jesus.

♦ **Proverbs 14:30a:** A tranquil heart is life to the body.

♦ **John 14:27:** Peace I leave with you, My peace I give unto you ... Let not your heart be troubled, nor let it be fearful.

Impending Death

♦ **Psalm 27:1-2:** The Lord is my light and my salvation; whom shall I fear? The Lord is the defense of my life; whom shall I dread: When evildoers came upon me to devour my flesh, my adversaries and my enemies, they stumbled and fell.

♦ **Psalm 91:14-16:** Because he has loved Me, therefore I will deliver him; I will set him securely on high because He has known My name. He will call upon Me, and I will answer him; I will be with him in trouble; I will rescue him, and honor him. With a long life I will satisfy him, and let him behold My salvation.

♦ **Psalm 118:16-17:** The right hand of the Lord is exalted; The right hand of the Lord does valiantly. I shall not die, but live, and tell of the works of the Lord.

♦ **Romans 8:2:** For the law of the Spirit of life in Christ Jesus has set you free from the law of sin and of death.

♦ **Romans 8:11:** But if the Spirit of Him who raised Jesus from the dead dwells in you, He who raised Christ Jesus from the dead will give life to your mortal bodies through His Spirit who indwells you.

♦ **Ephesians 6:2-3:** Honor your father and mother (which is the first commandment with a promise), that it may be well with you, and that you may live long on the earth.

Kidney and Urinary Tract Problems

♦ **Ezekiel 47:8-9:** (Speaking of the river of living water flowing from God's temple.) These waters pour out ... into the Dead Sea. And when they shall enter into the sea ... of putrid waters, the waters shall be healed and made fresh. ... And everything shall live wherever the river goes. (Amplified).

(Author's note: The Lord quickened me, when praying for urinary problems, to ask that the river of living water flow throughout the urinary tract to cleanse and heal.)

♦ **Revelation 22:1:** Then he showed me a river whose waters give life ... flowing out from the throne of God and of the Lamb. (Amplified).

♦ **John 7:37b-38:** If any man is thirsty, let him come to me and drink. He who believes in Me, as the Scripture said, "From his innermost being shall flow rivers of living water."

♦ **Exodus 23:25-26:** You shall serve the Lord your God, and He will bless your bread and your water; and I will remove sickness from your midst. ... I will fulfill the number of your days.

♦ **Mark 11:23:** (For Kidney Stones.) Truly I say to you, whosoever says to this mountain, "Be taken up and cast into the sea," and does not doubt in his heart, but believes that what he says is going to happen, it shall be granted to him.

♦ **Matthew 8:17b:** He Himself took our infirmities and carried away our diseases.

Malfunctioning of Organs or Glands
(Including Chemical or Hormonal Imbalances)

♦ **Psalm 139:14:** I will give thanks to Thee, for I am fearfully and wonderfully made; wonderful are Thy works, and my soul knows it very well.

♦ **Proverbs 4:20-22:** My son, give attention to my words; incline your ear to my sayings. Do not let them depart from your sight; keep them in the midst of your heart. For they are life to those who find them, and health (Lit. "medicine") to all their whole body.

♦ **1 Cor. 6:19-20:** Or do you not know that your body is a temple of the Holy Spirit who is in you, whom you have from God, and that you are not your own? For you have been bought with a price?

♦ **Romans 8:2:** For the law of the Spirit of life in Christ Jesus has set you free from the law of sin and of death. (We must release the law of the Spirit of life to take control of those parts of the body that are malfunctioning.)

♦ **Matthew 8:17b:** "He Himself took our infirmities, and carried away our diseases."

Muscle Diseases

♦ **Malachi 4:2:** But for you who fear My name the sun of righteousness will rise with healing in its wings; and you will go forth and skip about like calves from the stall.

♦ **Isaiah 40:29-31:** He gives strength to the weary, and to him who lacks might He increases power. Though youths grow weary and tired, and vigorous young men stumble badly, yet those who wait for the Lord will gain new strength; they will mount up with wings like eagles, they will run and not get tired, they will walk and not become weary.

♦ **Psalm 27:1-2:** The Lord is my light and my salvation; whom shall I fear? The Lord is the defense of my life; whom shall I dread? When evildoers came upon me to devour my flesh, my adversaries and my enemies, they stumbled and fell.

♦ **Psalm 18:29, 34:** For by Thee I can run upon a troop; and by my God I can leap over a wall. He trains my hands for battle, so that my arms can bend a bow of bronze.

♦ **Romans 8:2:** For the law of the Spirit of life in Christ Jesus has set you free from the law of sin and of death.

Nervous System and Emotional Illnesses

♦ **Proverbs 3:7-8:** Be not wise in your own eyes; reverently fear and worship the Lord, and turn away from evil. It shall be health to your nerves and sinews, and morrow and moistening to your bones. (Amplified)

♦ **Isaiah 53:4-5:** Surely He has borne our griefs – sickness, weakness and distress – and carried our sorrows and pain. ... He was wounded for our transgressions, He was bruised for our guilt and iniquities; the chastisement needful to obtain peace and well-being for us was upon Him, and with the stripes that wounded Him we are healed and made whole. (Amplified).

♦ **Psalm 116:8-9:** For Thou hast rescued my soul from death, my eyes from tears, my feet from stumbling. I shall walk before the Lord in the land of the living.

♦ **Isaiah 26:3:** Thou wilt keep him in perfect peace, whose mind is stayed on Thee; because he trusteth in Thee.

♦ **Psalm 138:7:** Though I walk in the midst of trouble, Thou wilt revive me.

♦ **Proverbs 4:20-22:** My son, give attention to my words; incline your ear to my sayings. Do not let them depart from your sight; keep them in the midst of your heart. For they are life to those who find them, and health (Lit. "medicine") to all their whole body.

♦ **Philippians 4:6-7:** Be anxious for nothing, but in everything by prayer and supplication with thanksgiving let your requests be made known to God. And the peace of God, which surpasses all comprehension, shall guard your hearts and your minds in Christ Jesus.

♦ **Isaiah 54:13-14:** And all your spiritual children (believers) shall be disciples – taught of the Lord and obedient to His will; and great shall be the peace and undisturbed composure of your children (believers). You shall establish yourself on righteousness ... You shall be far even from the thought of oppression or destruction, for you shall not fear; and from terror, for it shall not come near you. (Amplified).

♦ **John 14:27:** Peace I leave with you; My peace I give to you. ... Let not your heart be troubled; nor let it be afraid.

♦ **Romans 8:2:** For the law of the Spirit of life in Christ Jesus has set you free from the law of sin and of death.

Paralysis and Strokes

♦ **Romans 8:11:** But if the Spirit of Him who raised Jesus from the dead dwells in you, He who raised Christ Jesus from the dead will also give life to your mortal bodies through His Spirit who indwells you.

♦ **Romans 8:2:** For the law of the Spirit of life in Christ Jesus has set you free from the law of sin and of death.

♦ **Malachi 4:2:** But for you who fear My name the sun of righteousness will rise with healing in its wings; and you will go forth and skip about like calves from the stall.

♦ **Psalm 103:1-5:** Bless the Lord, O my soul, and all that is within me, bless His holy name. Bless the Lord, O my soul, and forget none of His benefits; who pardons all your iniquities; who heals all your diseases; who redeems your life from the pit; who crowns you with loving kindness and compassion; who satisfies your years with good things, so that your youth is renewed like the eagle.

♦ **Psalm 116:8-9:** For Thou hast rescued my soul from death, my eyes from tears, my feet from stumbling. I shall walk before the Lord in the land of the living.

♦ **1 Cor. 6:19-20:** Or do you not know that your body is a temple of the Holy Spirit who is in you, whom you have from God, and that you are not your own? For you have been bought with a price?

♦ **Isaiah 40:29-31:** He gives strength to the weary, and to him who lacks might He increases power. Though youths grow weary and tired, and vigorous young men stumble badly, yet those who wait for the Lord will gain new strength; they will mount up with wings like eagles, they will run and not get tired, they will walk and not become weary.

♦ **Psalm 118:16b-17:** The right hand of the Lord does valiantly. I shall not die, but live, and tell of the works of the Lord.

Protection from Communicable Diseases & Accidental Injuries

♦ **Psalm 91:1-13:** He who dwells in the shelter of the Most High will abide in the shadow of the Almighty. I will say to the Lord, "My refuge and my fortress, my God, in whom I trust!" For it is He who delivers you from the snare of the trapper, and from the deadly pestilence. He will cover you with His pinions, and under His wings you may seek refuge; His faithfulness is a shield and bulwark. You will not be afraid of the terror by night, or of the arrow that flies by day; of the pestilence that stalks in darkness, or the destruction that lays waste at noon. A thousand may fall at your side and ten thousand at your right hand; but it shall not approach you. You will only look on with your eyes, and see the recompense of the wicked. For you have made the Lord, my refuge, even the Most High, your dwelling place. No evil will befall you, nor will any plague come near your tent. For He will give His angels charge concerning you, to guard you in all your ways. They will bear you up in their hands, lest you strike your foot against a stone. You will tread upon the lion and cobra, the young lion and the serpent you will trample down.

♦ **Luke 10:19:** Behold, I have given you authority to tread upon serpents and scorpions, and over all the power of the enemy, and nothing shall injure you.

♦ **Isaiah 54:17a:** No weapon that is formed against you shall prosper.

♦ **Romans 8:2:** For the law of the Spirit of life in Christ Jesus has set you free from the law of sin and of death.

Reproductive System Problems

♦ **Exodus 23:25-26:** But you shall serve the Lord your God, and He will bless your bread and your water; and I will remove sickness from your midst. There shall be no one miscarrying or barren in your land; I will fulfill the number of your days.

♦ **Deut. 7:14-15:** You shall be blessed above all peoples; there shall be no male or female barren among you or among your cattle. And the Lord will remove from you all sickness.

♦ **Psalm 113:9:** He maketh the barren woman to keep house, and to be a joyful mother of children. (KJV).

♦ **Deut. 28:2-4a:** And all these blessings shall come upon you and overtake you, if you will obey the Lord your God. Blessed shall you be in the city, and blessed shall you be in the country. Blessed shall be the offspring of your body.

♦ **2 Tim. 2:15:** But women shall be preserved through the bearing of children if they continue in faith and love and sanctity with self-restraint.

♦ **Romans 8:2:** For the law of the Spirit of life in Christ Jesus has set you free from the law of sin and of death.

Stomach & Intestinal Problems

♦ **Exodus 23:25:** But you shall serve the Lord your God, and He will bless your bread and your water; and I will remove sickness from your midst.

♦ **Psalm 107:17-20:** Fools because of their rebellious way and because of their iniquities, were afflicted. Their soul abhorred all kinds of food; and they drew near to the gates of death. They cried out to the Lord in their trouble; He saved them out of their distresses. He sent His word and healed them, and delivered them from their destructions.

♦ **John 7:38:** He that believeth on me, as the Scripture hath said, out of his belly shall flow rivers of living water. (KJV).

♦ **Psalm 103:2-5:** Bless the Lord, O my soul, and forget none of His benefits: Who forgiveth all thine iniquities; who healeth all thy diseases; who redeemeth thy life from destruction; who crowneth thee with lovingkindness and tender mercies; who satisfieth thy mouth with good things, so that thy youth is renewed like the eagle's.

Tooth Problems

- **Psalm 3:7b-8:** Thou hast shattered the teeth of the wicked. Salvation belongs to the Lord; Thy blessing be upon Thy people! (If it's the teeth of the wicked that are broken, God's people should be able to claim the blessing of healthy teeth.)

- **Psalm 103:5:** Who satisfieth thy mouth with good things, so that thy youth is renewed like the eagle's. (KJV).

- **Romans 8:11:** But if the Spirit of Him who raised Jesus from the dead dwells in you, He who raised Christ Jesus from the dead will also give life to your mortal bodies through His Spirit who indwells you.

Tuberculosis and Other Lung Disease

- **Galatians 3:13:** Christ redeemed us from the curse of the Law, having become a curse for us. (Tuberculosis / Consumption is listed specifically as part of the curse of the Law in Deut. 28:22.)

- **Psalm 27:1-2:** The Lord is my light and my salvation; whom shall I fear? The Lord is the defense of my life; whom shall I dread? When evildoers came upon me to devour my flesh, my adversaries and my enemies, they stumbled and fell.

♦ **Psalm 107:18-20:** Their soul abhorred all kinds of food; and they drew near to the gates of death. They cried out to the Lord in their trouble; He saved them out of their distresses. He sent His word and healed them, and delivered them from their destructions.

♦ **Psalm 103:2-5:** Bless the Lord, O my soul, and forget none of His benefits; who pardons all your iniquities; who heals all your diseases; who redeems your life from the pit; who crowns you with loving kindness and compassion; who satisfies your years with good things, so that your youth is renewed like the eagle.

♦ **Acts 17:25b:** He Himself gives to all life and breath and all things.

♦ **Genesis 2:7:** Then the Lord God formed man of dust from the ground, and breathed into his nostrils the breath of life.

♦ **Matthew 8:16-17:** And when evening had come, they brought to Him many that were demon-possessed; and He cast out the spirits with a word, and healed all who were ill in order that what was spoken through Isaiah the prophet might be fulfilled, saying, "He Himself took our infirmities, and carried away our diseases."

Venereal Diseases and Other Sickness
or Injury Resulting from a Known Sin

♦ **Ps. 107:17-20:** Fools because of their rebellious way
and because of their iniquities, were afflicted. Their
soul abhorred all kinds of food; and they drew near to
the gates of death. They cried out to the Lord in their
trouble; He saved them out of their distresses. He
sent His word and healed them, and delivered them
from their destructions.

♦ **Isaiah 53:4-5:** Surely He has borne our griefs –
sickness, weakness and distress – and carried our
sorrows and pain. ... He was wounded for our
transgressions, He was bruised for our guilt and
iniquities; the chastisement needful to obtain peace
and well-being for us was upon Him, and with the
stripes that wounded Him we are healed and made
whole. (Amplified).

♦ **Matthew 9:2-7:** And behold, they were bringing to
Him a paralytic, lying on a bed; and Jesus seeing their
faith said to the paralytic, "Take courage, My son,
your sins are forgiven." And behold, some of the
scribes said to themselves. "This fellow blasphemes."
And Jesus knowing their thoughts said, "Why are you
thinking evil in your hearts? For which is easier to
say, 'Your sins are forgiven' or to say, 'Rise and

walk?' But in order that you may know that the Son of Man has authority on earth to forgive sins" -- then He said to the paralytic, "Rise, take up your bed and go home." And he rose and went to his home.

♦ **Galatians 3:13:** Christ redeemed us from the curse of the Law, having become a curse for us.

♦ **John 8:36:** If the Son therefore shall make you free, ye shall be free indeed.

♦ **James 5:14-15:** Is anyone among you sick? Let him call for the elders of the church, and let them pray over him, anointing him with oil in the name of the Lord; and the prayer offered in faith will restore the one who is sick, and the Lord will raise him up, and if he has committed sins, they will be forgiven him.

♦ **Romans 8:5-6:** For those who are according to the flesh set their minds on the things of the flesh, but those who are according to the Spirit, the things of the Spirit. For the mind set on the flesh is death, but the mind set on the Spirit is life and peace.

♦ **Romans 8:2:** For the law of the Spirit of life in Christ Jesus has set you free from the law of sin and of death.

Weakness

♦ **Isaiah 40:29-31:** He gives strength to the weary, and to him who lacks might He increases power. Though youths grow weary and tired, and vigorous young men stumble badly, yet those who wait for the Lord will gain new strength; they will mount up with wings like eagles, they will run and not get tired, they will walk and not become weary.

♦ **Psalm 18:1-2:** I will love Thee, O Lord, my strength. The Lord is my rock, and my fortress, and my deliverer; my God, my strength in whom I trust. (KJV).

♦ **Psalm 68:28a:** Your God has commanded your strength.

♦ **Nehemiah 8:10:** Then he said to them, "Go, eat of the fat, drink of the sweet, and send portions to him who has nothing prepared; for this day is holy to our Lord. Do not be grieved, for the joy of the Lord is our strength.

♦ **2 Timothy 1:7:** For God hath not given us the spirit of fear; but of power, and of love, and of a sound mind. (KJV).

♦ **Philippians 4:13:** I can do all things through Him who strengthens me.

♦ **Isaiah 41:10:** Do not fear, for I am with you; do not anxiously look about you, for I am your God. I will strengthen you, surely I will help you, surely I will uphold you with My righteous right hand.

General Healing Scriptures

♦ **Exodus 15:26:** If you will give earnest heed to the voice of the Lord your God, and do what is right in His sight, and give ear to His commandments, and keep all His statutes, I will put none of the diseases on you which I have put on the Egyptians; for I, the Lord, am your healer (physician).

♦ **Proverbs 4:20-22:** My son, give attention to my words; incline your ear to my sayings. Do not let them depart from your sight; keep them in the midst of your heart. For they are life to those who find them, and health (Lit. "medicine") to all their whole body.

♦ **3 John 2:** Beloved, I pray that in all respects you may prosper and be in good health, just as your soul prospers.

♦ **Psalm 103:1-5:** Bless the Lord, O my soul, and all that is within me, bless His holy name. Bless the

Lord, O my soul, and forget none of His benefits; who pardons all your iniquities; who heals all your diseases; who redeems your life from the pit; who crowns you with loving kindness and compassion; who satisfies your years with good things, so that your youth is renewed like the eagle.

♦ **Isaiah 53:4-5:** Surely He has borne our griefs – sickness, weakness and distress – and carried our sorrows and pain. ... He was wounded for our transgressions, He was bruised for our guilt and iniquities; the chastisement needful to obtain peace and well-being for us was upon Him, and with the stripes that wounded Him we are healed and made whole. (Amplified).

♦ **1 Peter 2:24:** And He Himself bore our sins in His body on the cross, that we might die to sin and live to righteousness; for by His wounds you were healed.

♦ **Matthew 8:16-17:** And when evening had come, they brought to Him many that were demon-possessed; and He cast out the spirits with a word, and healed all who were ill in order that what was spoken through Isaiah the prophet might be fulfilled, saying, "He Himself took our infirmities, and carried away our diseases."

♦ **Psalm 41:1-3:** How blessed is he who considers the helpless; the Lord will deliver him in a day of trouble. The Lord will protect him, and keep him alive, and he shall be called blessed upon the earth; and do not give him over to the desire of his enemies. The Lord will sustain him upon his sickbed; in his illness, Thou dost restore him to health.

♦ **John 14:13-14:** And what ever you ask in My name, that will I do, that the Father may be glorified in the son. If you ask Me anything in My name, I will do it.

♦ **1 John 5:14-15:** And this is the confidence which we have before Him, that if we ask anything according to His will, He hears us. And if we know that He hears us in whatever we ask, we know that we have the requests which we have asked from Him.

♦ **Mark 11:22b-25:** Have faith in God. Truly I say to you, whoever says to this mountain, "Be taken up and cast into the sea," and does not doubt in his heart, but believes that what he says is going to happen, it shall be granted him. Therefore, I say to you all things for which you pray and ask, believe that you have received them, and they shall be granted you. And whenever you stand praying, forgive, if you have anything against anyone; so that your Father also who is in heaven may forgive you your transgressions.

♦ **Galatians 3:13:** Christ redeemed us from the curse of the Law, having become a curse for us.

♦ **Romans 8:11:** But if the Spirit of Him who raised Jesus from the dead dwells in you, He who raised

Christ Jesus from the dead will also give life to your mortal bodies through His Spirit who indwells you.

- **Romans 8:2:** For the law of the Spirit of life in Christ Jesus has set you free from the law of sin and of death.

- **Exodus 23:25-26:** But you shall serve the Lord your God, and He will bless your bread and your water; and I will remove sickness from your midst. ... I will fulfill the number of your days.

- **Jeremiah 30:17:** For I will restore you to health, and I will heal you of your wounds, declares the Lord.

- **Romans 8:31-32:** What shall we then say to these things? If God be for us, who can be against us? He that spared not His own Son, but delivered Him up for us all, how shall He not with Him also freely give us all things? (KJV).

About the Author

Sandra Conner has been teaching God's Word and serving in ministry since she was fifteen years old. In 1975, the Lord baptized her in the Holy Spirit, and her work for the kingdom of God took on a deeper dimension and became more widespread. Since that time, the Lord has used Sandra to teach His anointed Word in meetings and seminars for many churches and Christian organizations, as well as through various media channels, including radio, television, and the numerous books and articles that she writes.

She and her husband Richard founded Healing Streams Ministries, and for twenty-two years had the privilege of working together in the Lord's work. They led home Bible studies, counseled individuals and families in need of healing for relationships, and ministered through the Word and the gifts of the Holy Spirit to help hurting people receive healing and deliverance from the Lord. Richard went to be with the Lord in 2002, and Sandra continued the ministry for many years. In 2011, she founded Radical About Jesus Ministries and added online teaching to her work, reaching thousands of people around the world through the "Healing From Jesus" website and the ministry YouTube channel.

To contact Sandra personally or for ministry engagements, e-mail her at the following address. Include Sandra's name in the subject line.

radicalaboutjesus@gmail .com

For more contact information, please turn the page.

Readers can also connect with Sandra
online at the following sites:

Radical About Jesus Ministries YouTube Channel
and
healingfromjesus.wordpress.com

Find other inspirational books by Sandra
(both fiction and non-fiction)
at Amazon.com

Made in United States
North Haven, CT
23 June 2024

53976840R10102